MAKEUP FACE CHARTS

Makeup makes everything **BETTER**

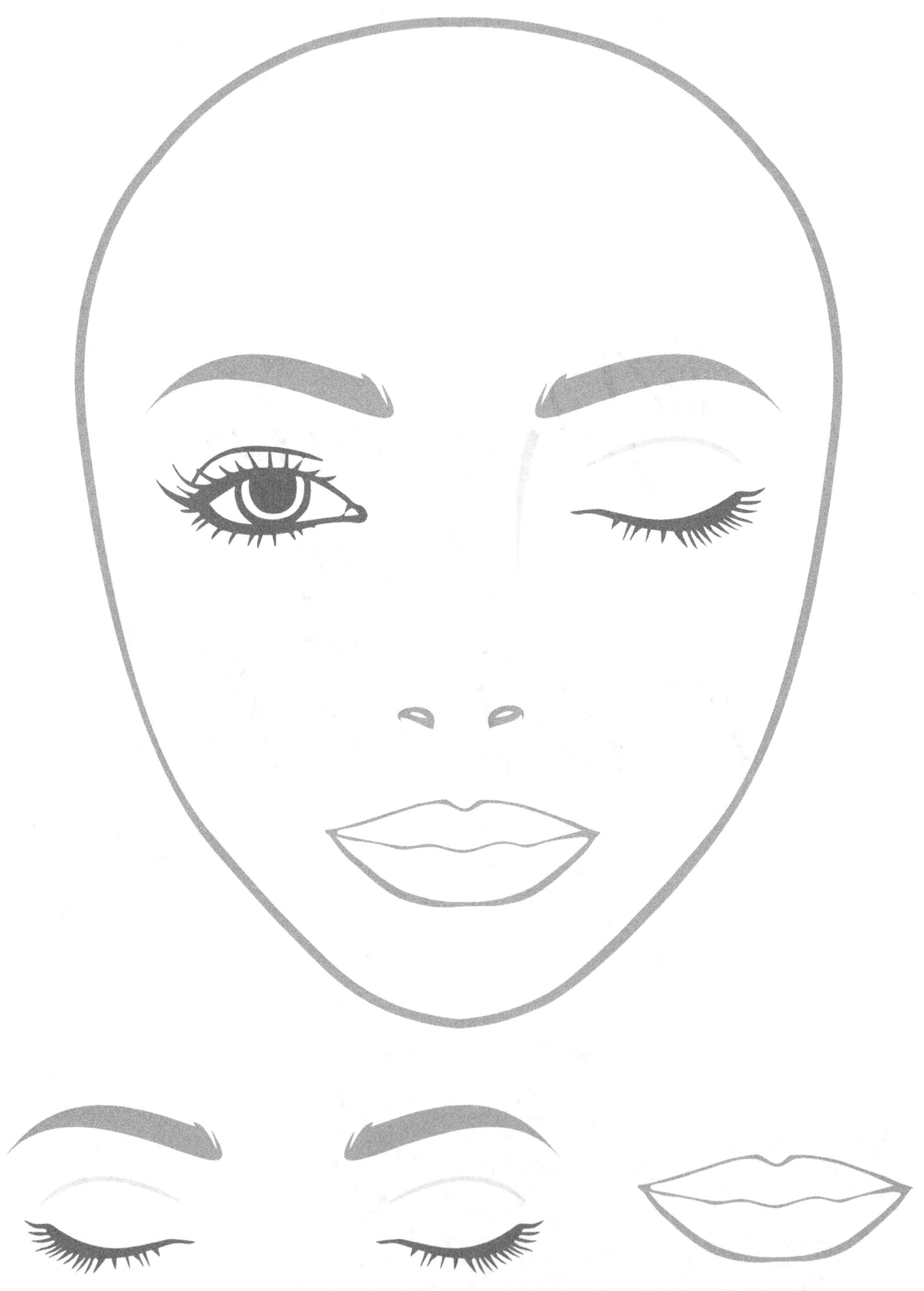

LOOK NAME ________________________ FOR: ________________________

○ Daytime   ○ Evening

FACE

Moisturizer

____

Primer

____

Powder

____

Highlight/Blush

____

Concealer

____

Foundation

____

Contour

____

EYES

Brows

____

Eyelid

____

Liner

____

Crease

____

Mascara

LIPS

Liner

____

Lip Color

____

Gloss

____

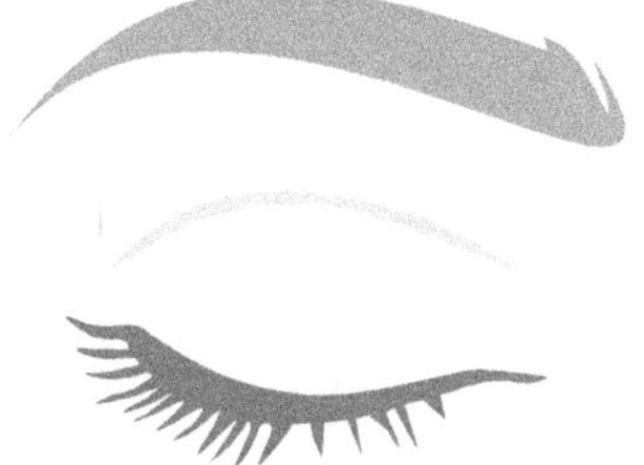
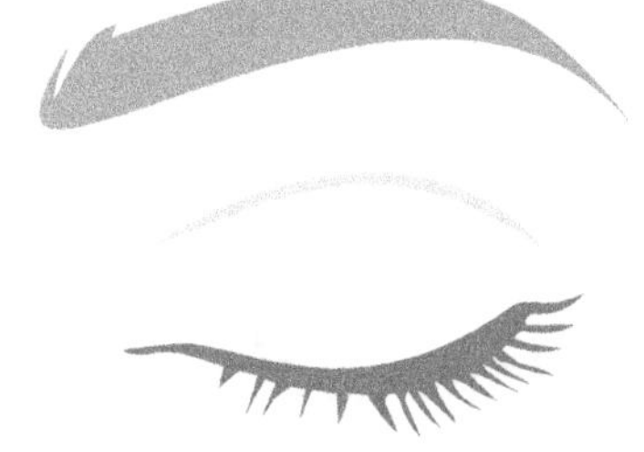
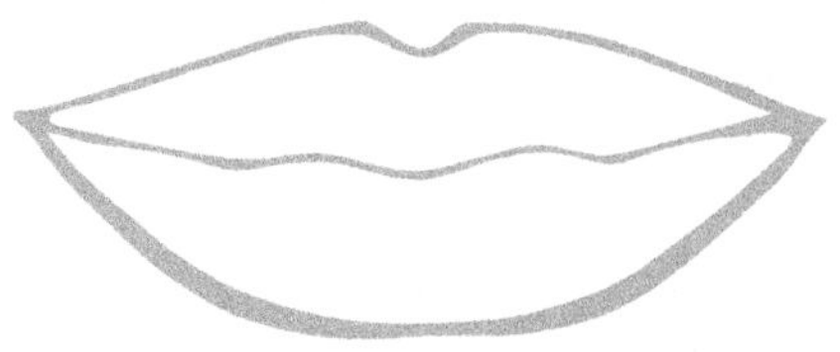

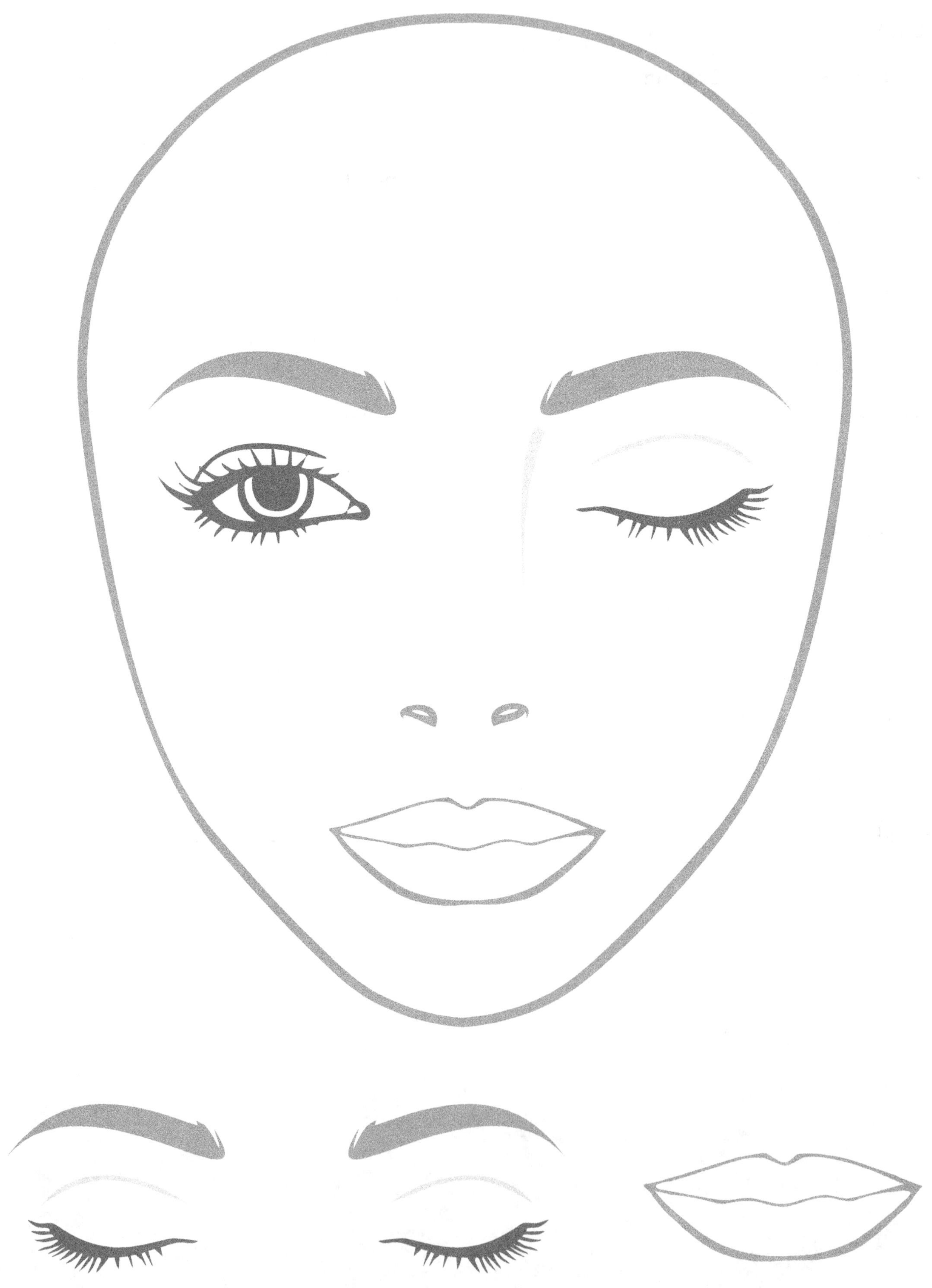

LOOK NAME _______________________ FOR: _______________________

◯ Daytime   ◯ Evening

FACE

Moisturizer

____

Primer

____

Powder

____

Highlight/Blush

____

Concealer

____

Foundation

____

Contour

____

EYES

Brows

____

Eyelid

____

Liner

____

Crease

____

Mascara

LIPS

Liner

____

Lip Color

____

Gloss

____

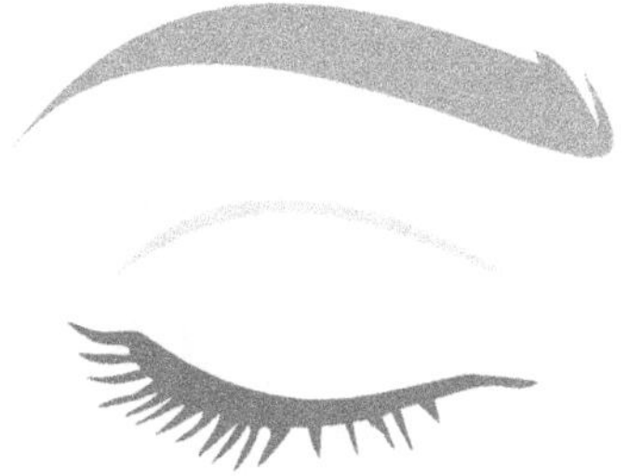
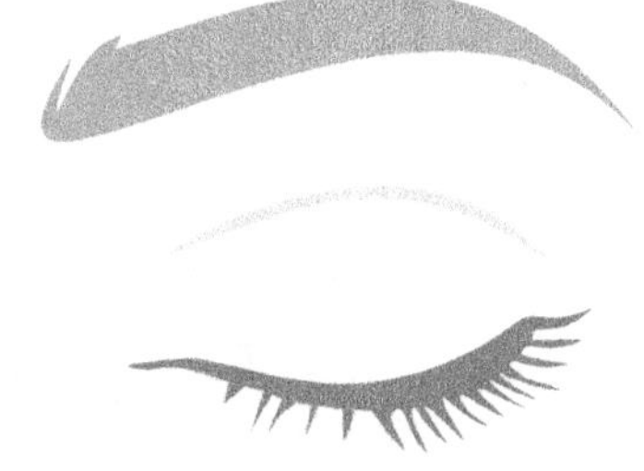
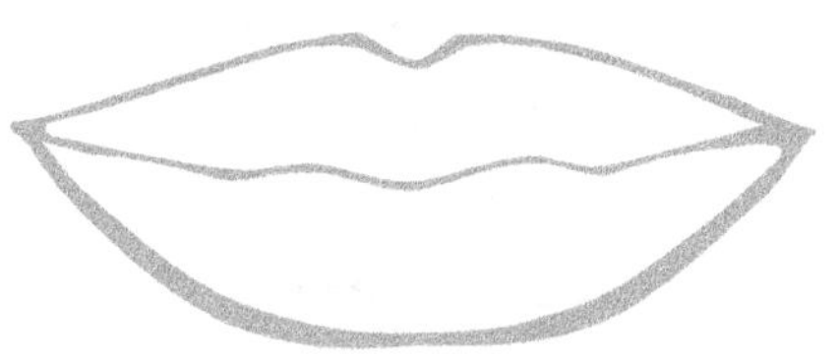

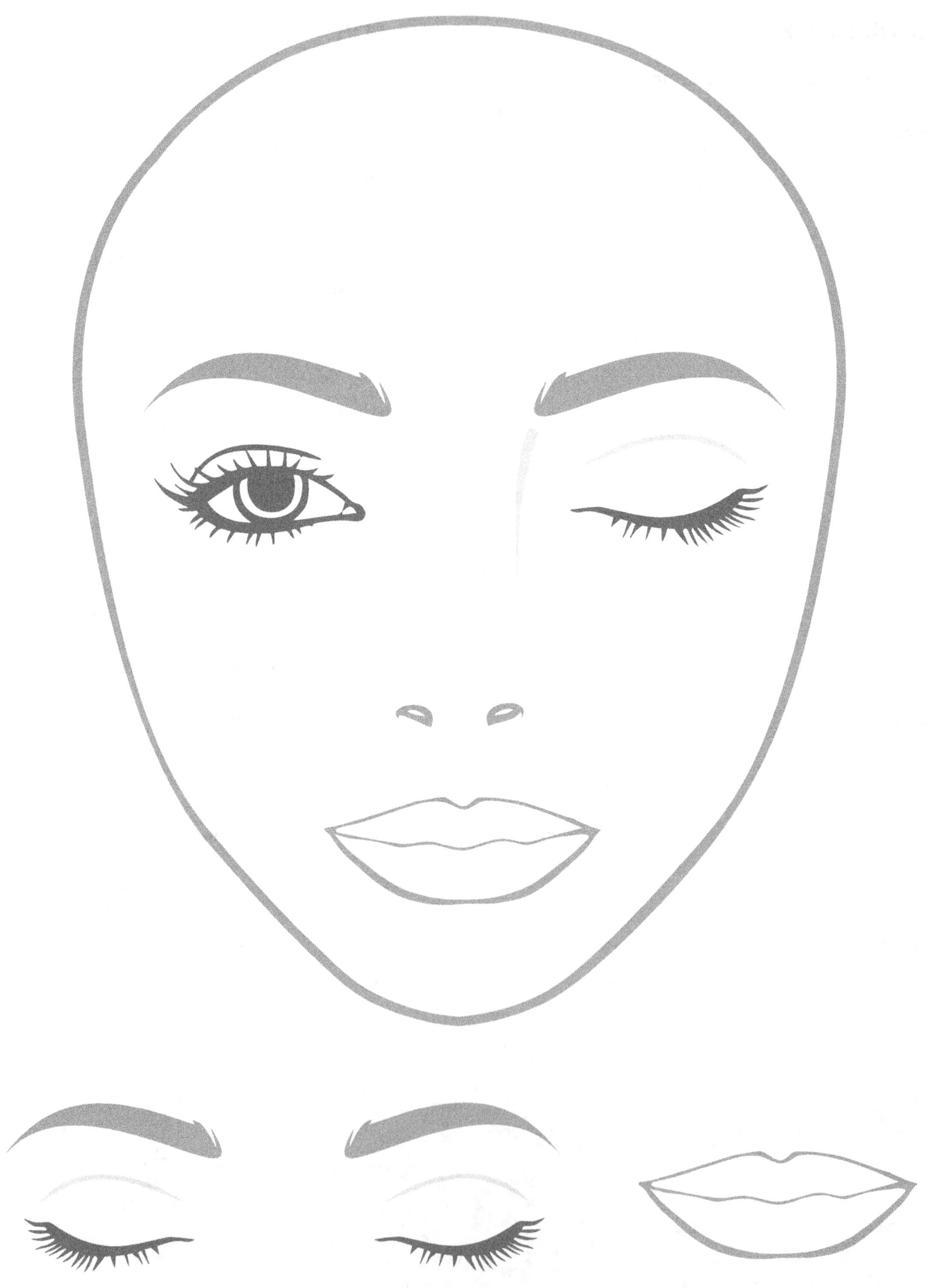

LOOK NAME ______________________________ **FOR:** ______________________

◯ Daytime   ◯ Evening

FACE

Moisturizer

____

Primer

____

Powder

____

Highlight/Blush

____

Concealer

____

Foundation

____

Contour

____

EYES

Brows

____

Eyelid

____

Liner

____

Crease

____

Mascara

____

LIPS

Liner

____

Lip Color

____

Gloss

____

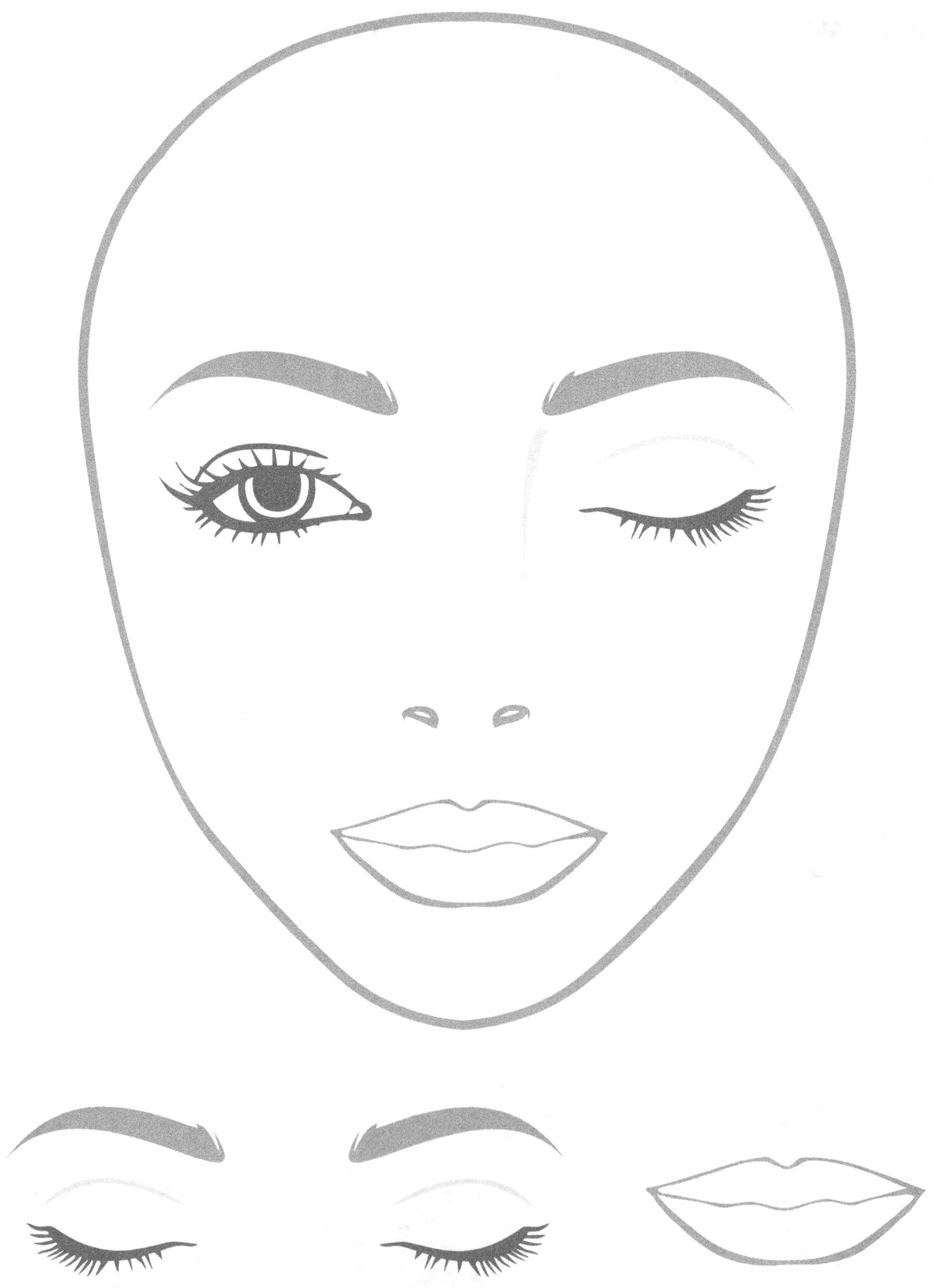

LOOK NAME _________________________   **FOR:** _________________________

◯ Daytime   ◯ Evening

FACE

Moisturizer

____

Primer

____

Powder

____

Highlight/Blush

____

Concealer

____

Foundation

____

Contour

____

EYES

Brows

____

Eyelid

____

Liner

____

Crease

____

Mascara

____

LIPS

Liner

____

Lip Color

____

Gloss

____

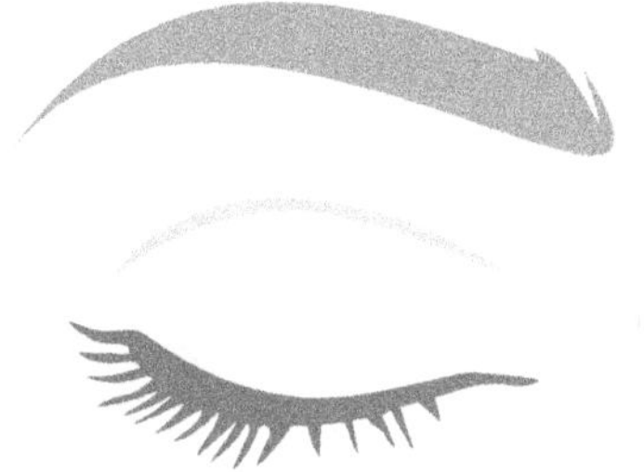
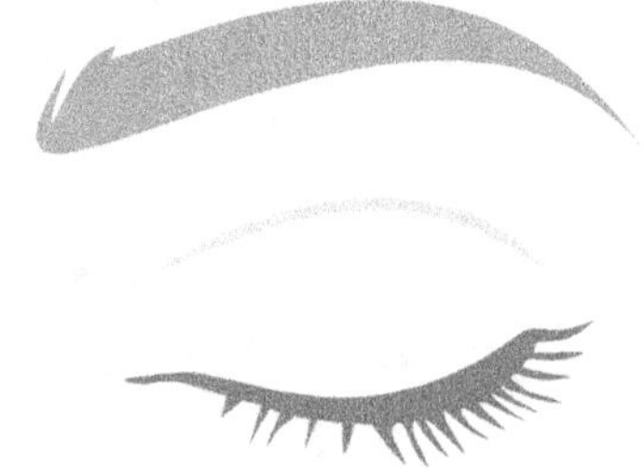
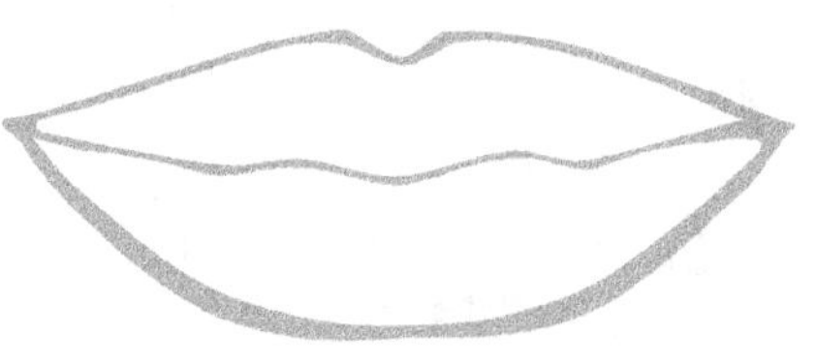

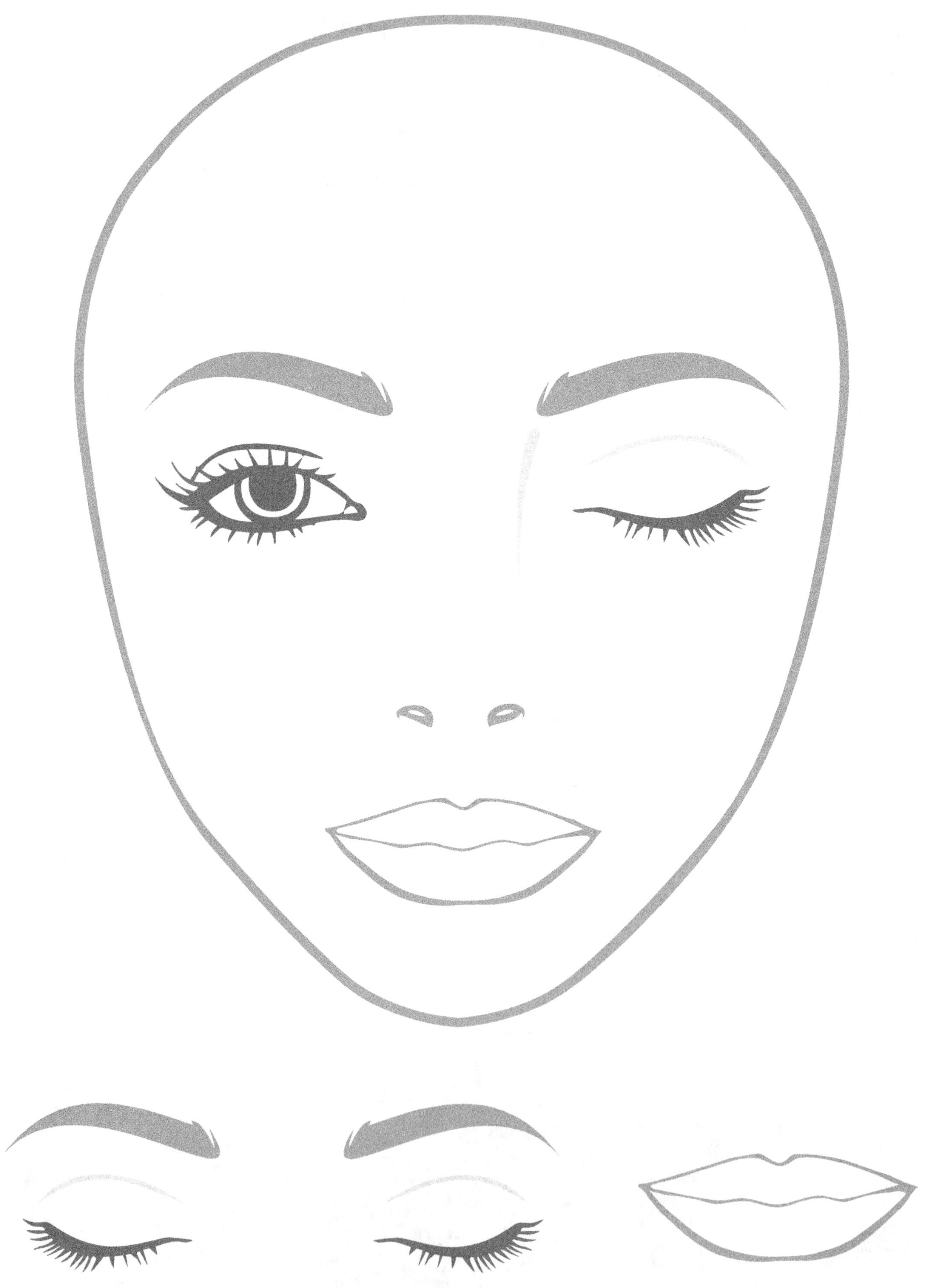

LOOK NAME _______________________   FOR: _______________________

○ Daytime   ○ Evening

FACE

Moisturizer

____

Primer

____

Powder

____

Highlight/Blush

____

Concealer

____

Foundation

____

Contour

____

EYES

Brows

____

Eyelid

____

Liner

____

Crease

____

Mascara

____

LIPS

Liner

____

Lip Color

____

Gloss

____

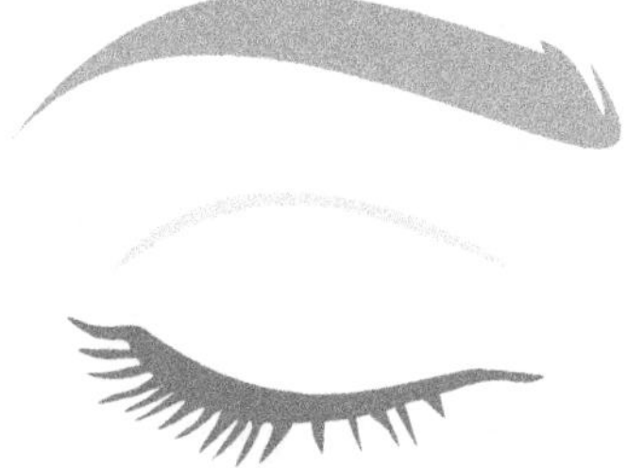
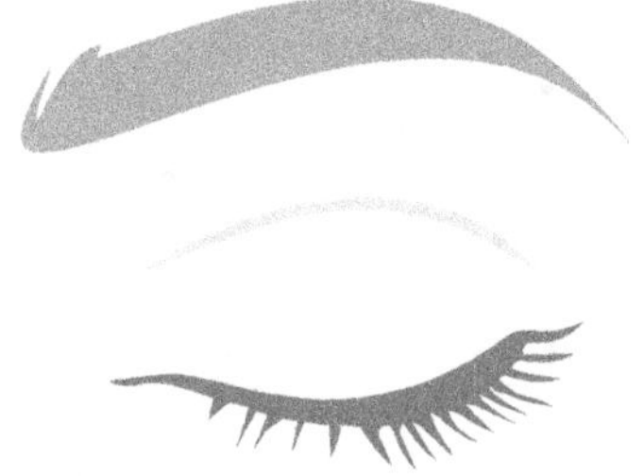
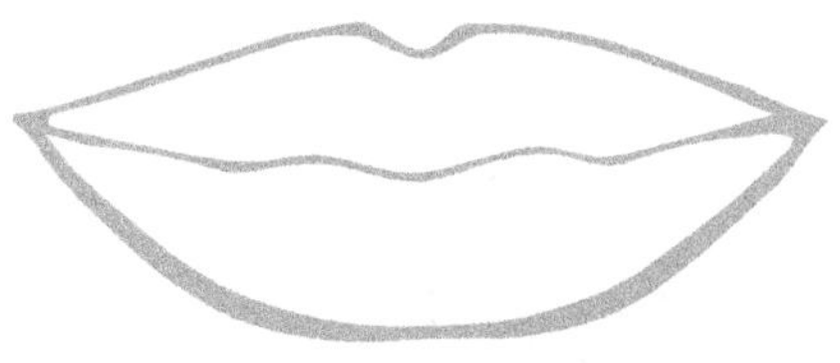

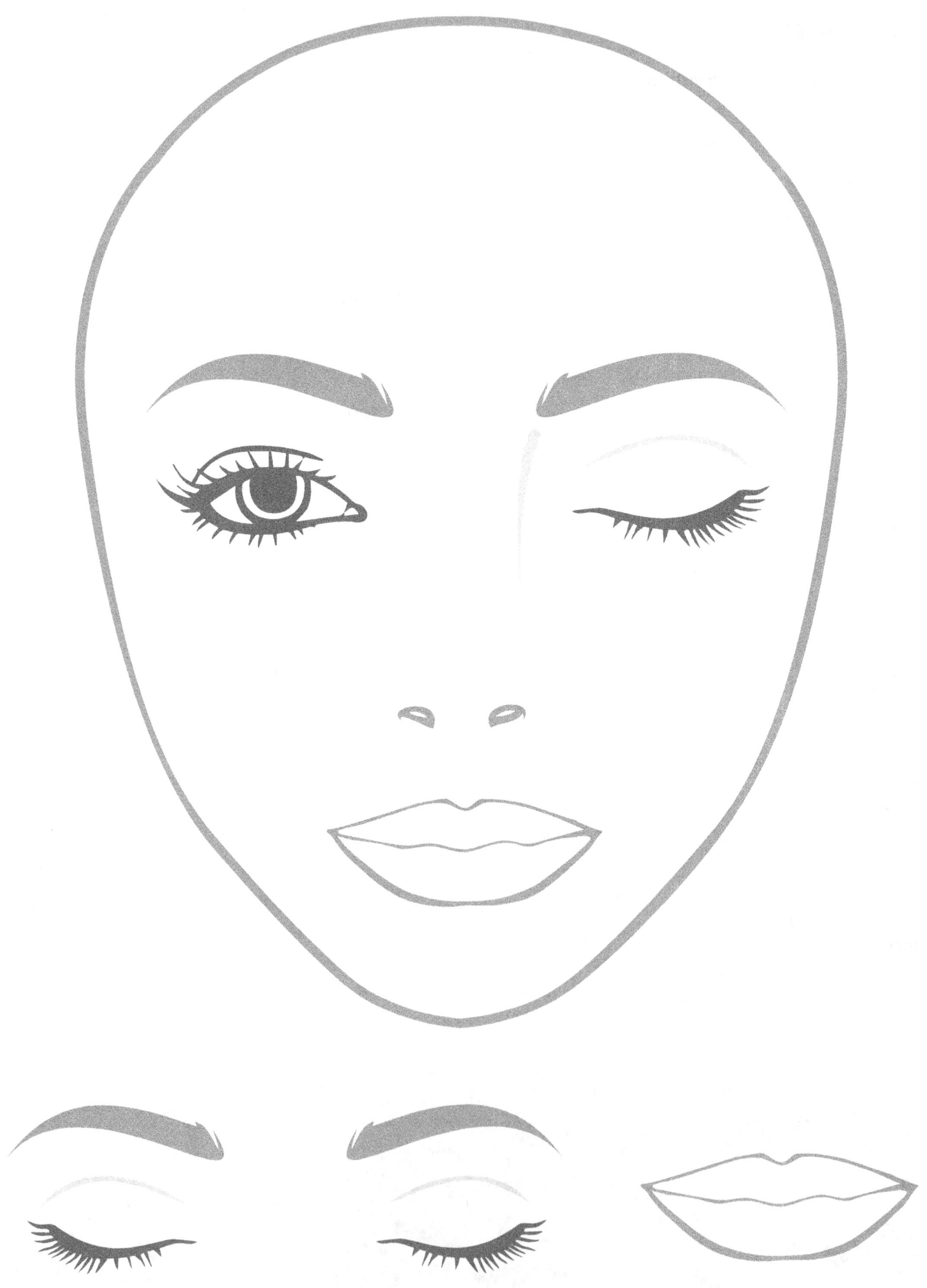

LOOK NAME _________________________ **FOR:** _________________________

◯ Daytime   ◯ Evening

FACE

Moisturizer

____

Primer

____

Powder

____

Highlight/Blush

____

Concealer

____

Foundation

____

Contour

____

EYES

Brows

____

Eyelid

____

Liner

____

Crease

____

Mascara

____

LIPS

Liner

____

Lip Color

____

Gloss

____

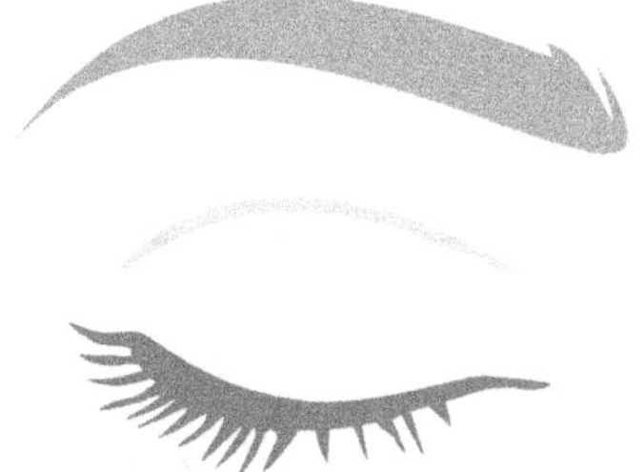
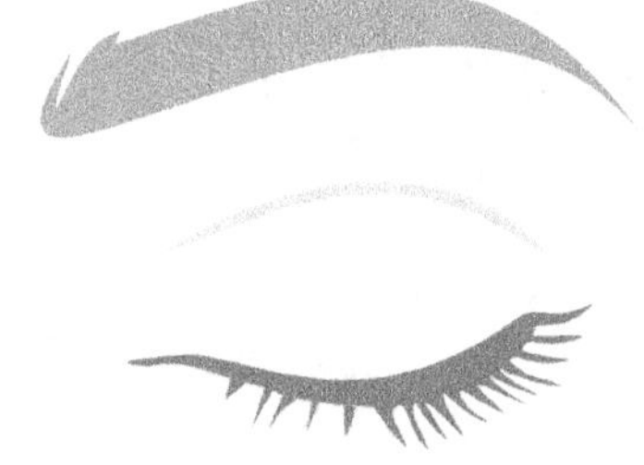
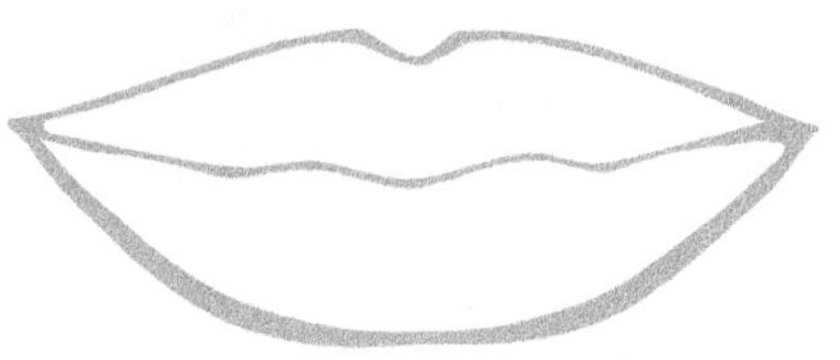

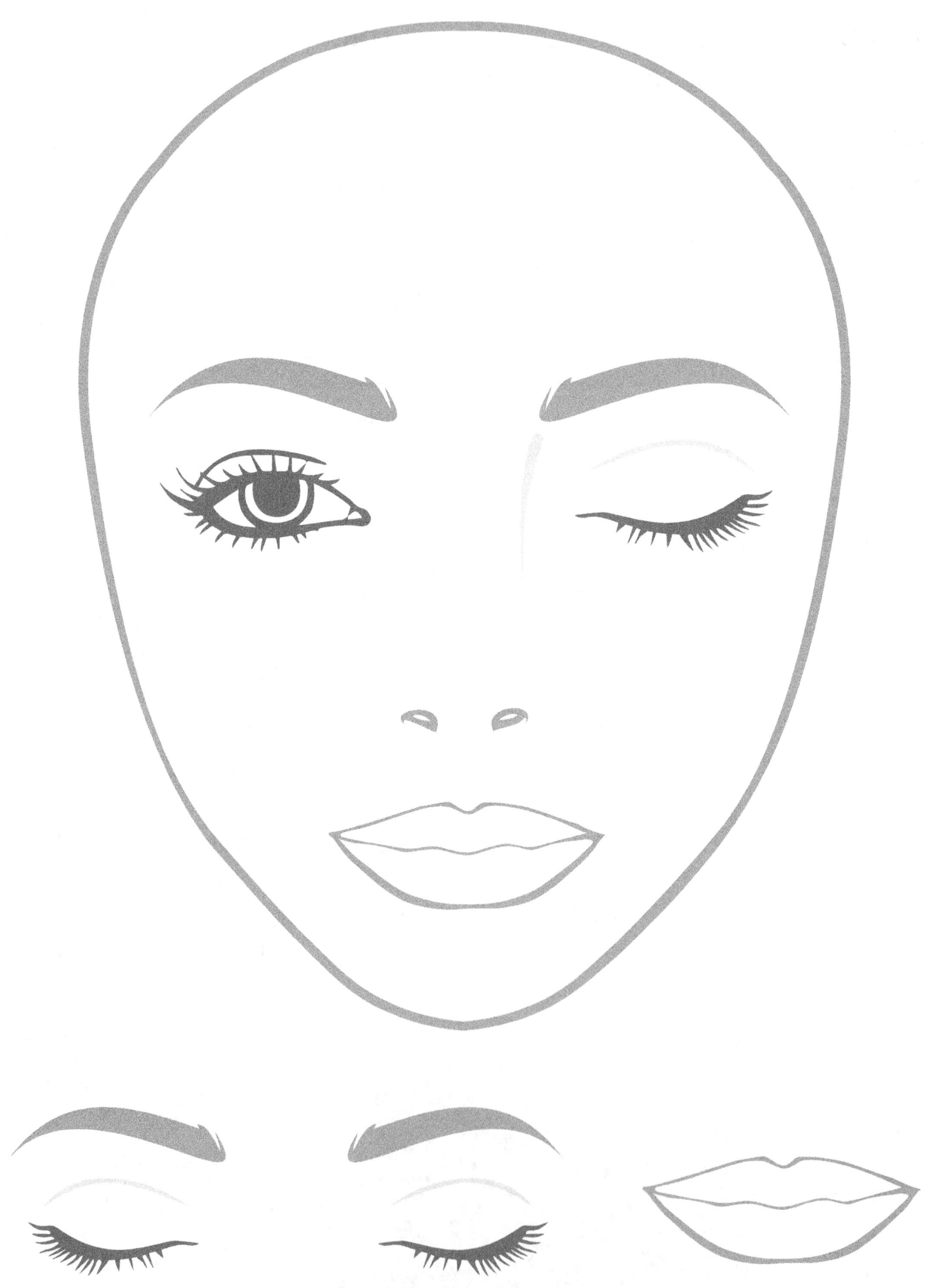

LOOK NAME _______________________ **FOR:** _______________________

◯ Daytime   ◯ Evening

FACE

Moisturizer

____

Primer

____

Powder

____

Highlight/Blush

____

Concealer

____

Foundation

____

Contour

____

EYES

Brows

____

Eyelid

____

Liner

____

Crease

____

Mascara

____

LIPS

Liner

____

Lip Color

____

Gloss

____

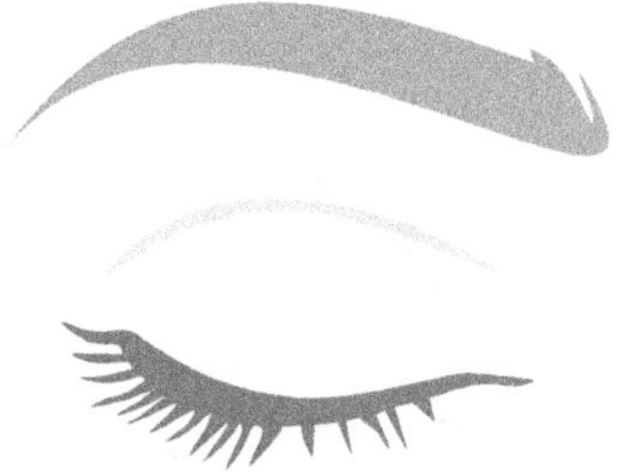
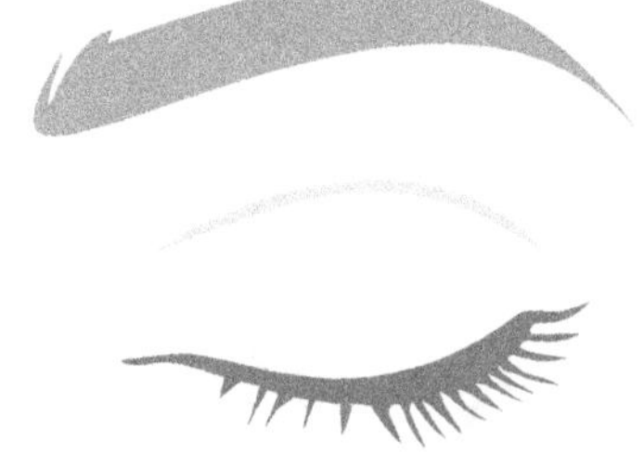
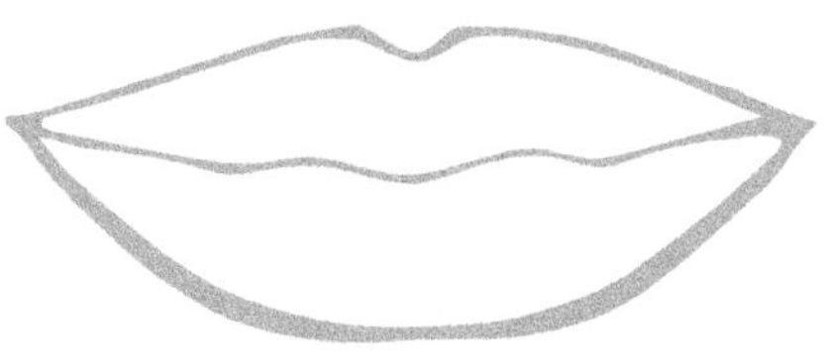

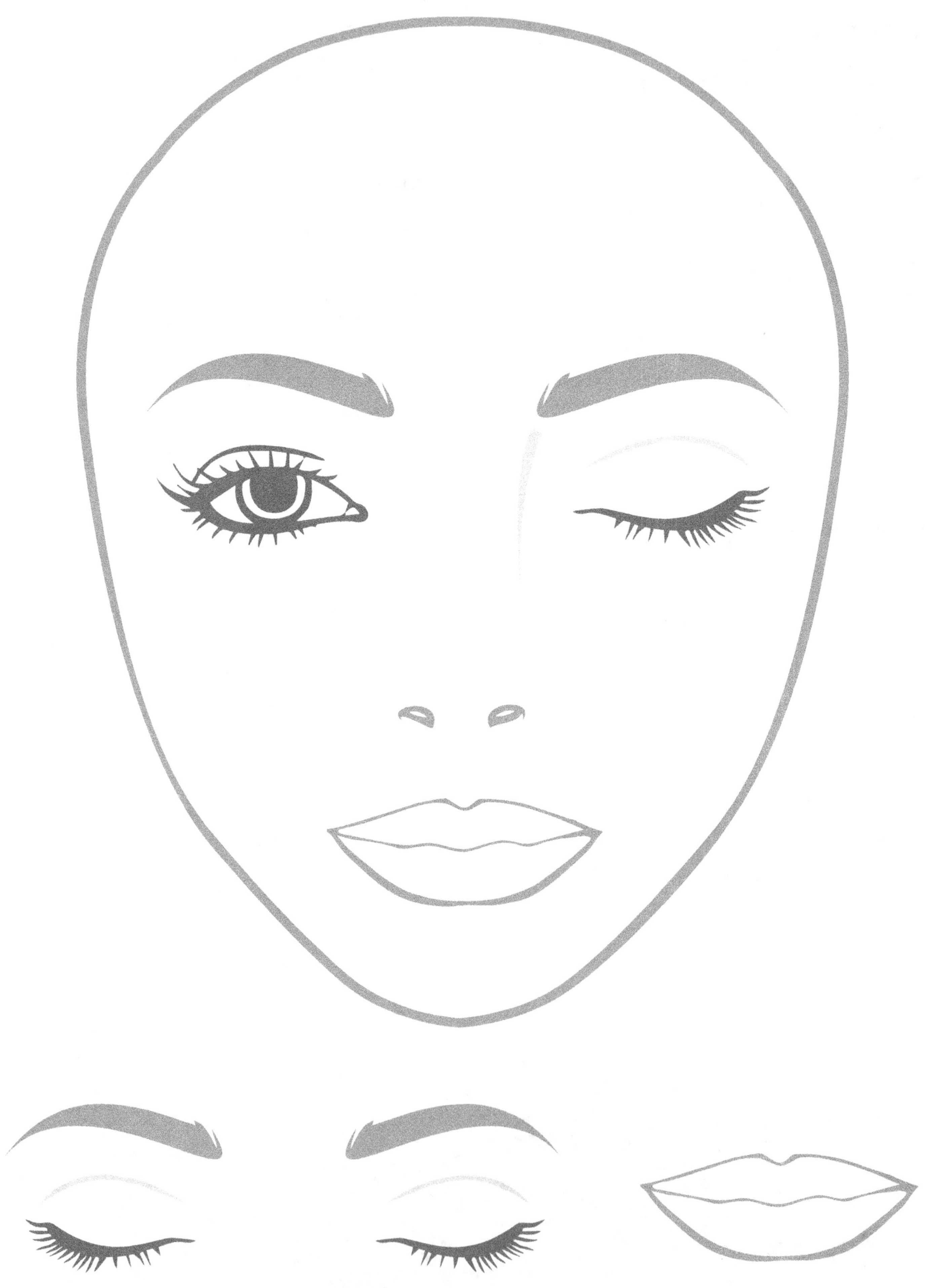

LOOK NAME _______________________ FOR: _______________________

○ Daytime   ○ Evening

FACE

Moisturizer

____

Primer

____

Powder

____

Highlight/Blush

____

Concealer

____

Foundation

____

Contour

____

EYES

Brows

____

Eyelid

____

Liner

____

Crease

____

Mascara

____

LIPS

Liner

____

Lip Color

____

Gloss

____

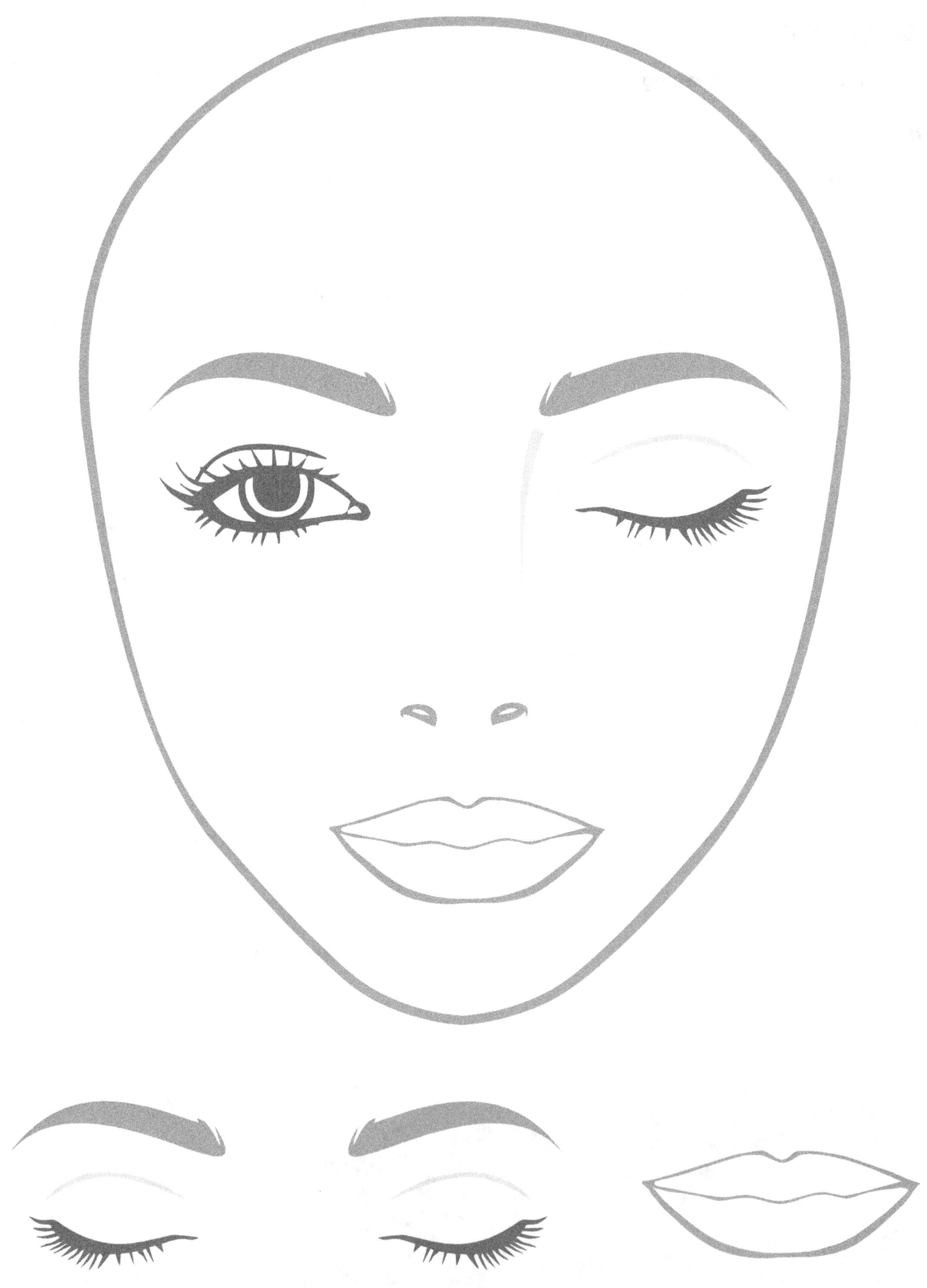

LOOK NAME ______________________   FOR: ______________________

○ Daytime   ○ Evening

FACE

Moisturizer

____

Primer

____

Powder

____

Highlight/Blush

____

Concealer

____

Foundation

____

Contour

____

EYES

Brows	Crease

____

Eyelid	Mascara

____

Liner

____

LIPS

Liner

____

Lip Color

____

Gloss

____

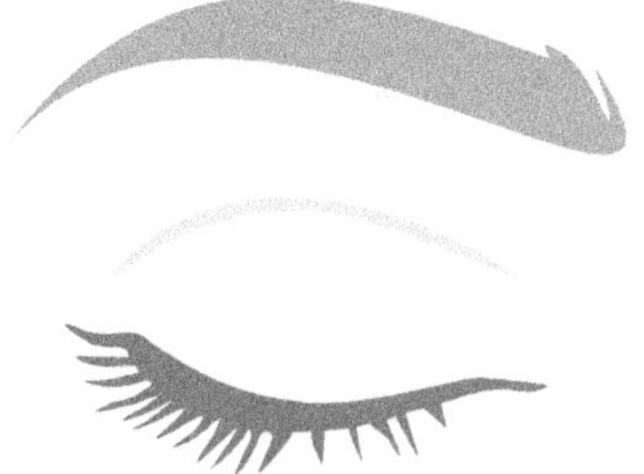

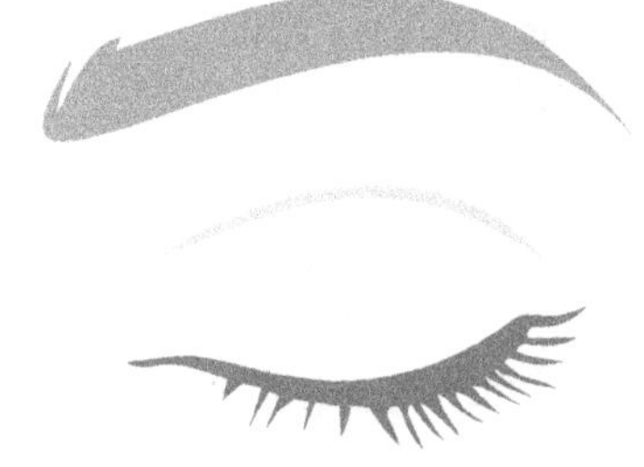

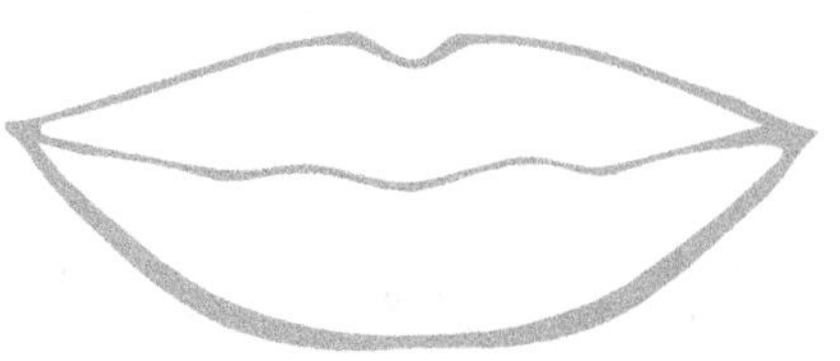

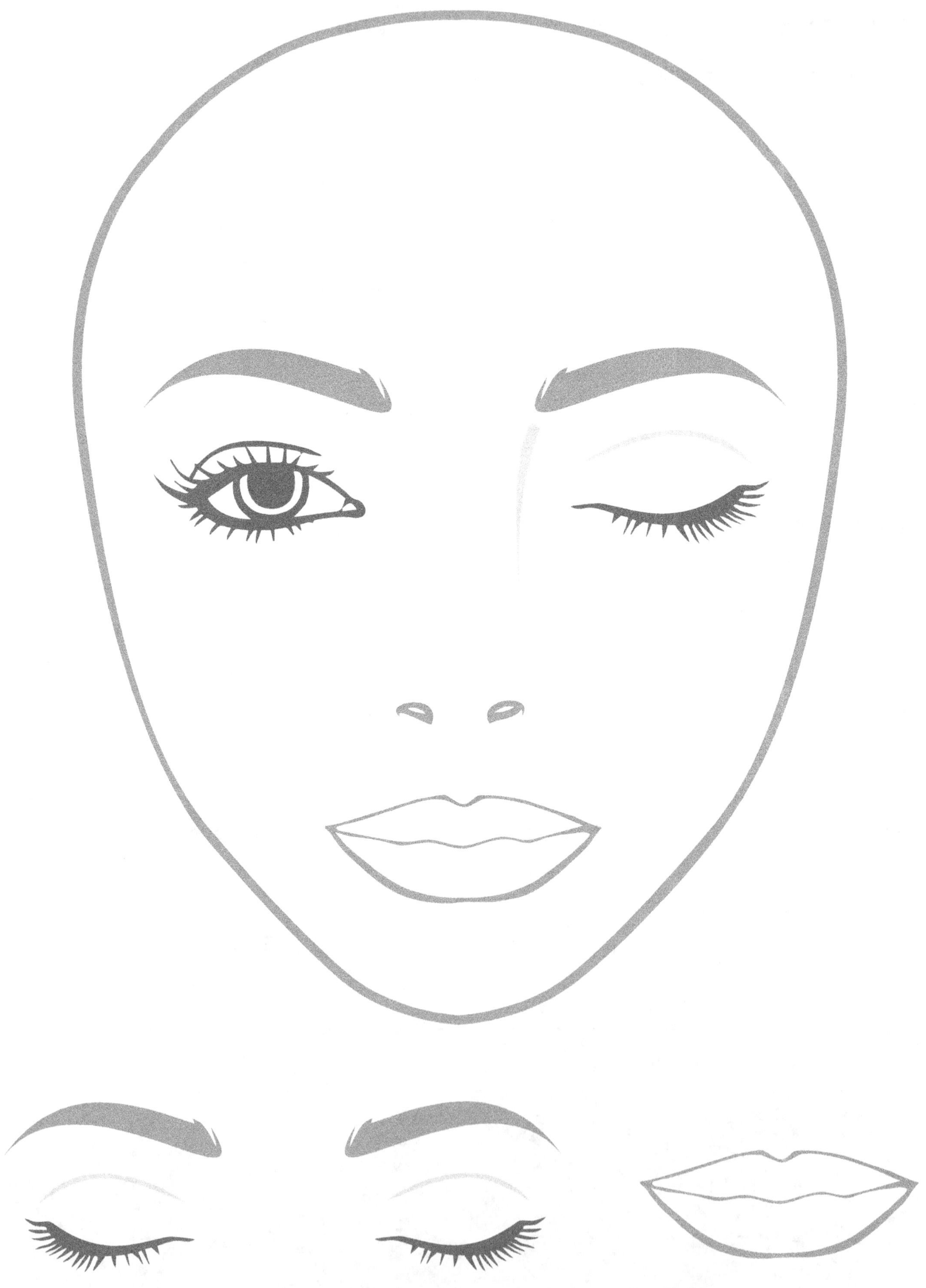

◯ Daytime   ◯ Evening

FACE

Moisturizer

____

Primer

____

Powder

____

Highlight/Blush

____

Concealer

____

Foundation

____

Contour

____

EYES

Brows

____

Eyelid

____

Liner

____

Crease

____

Mascara

____

LIPS

Liner

____

Lip Color

____

Gloss

____

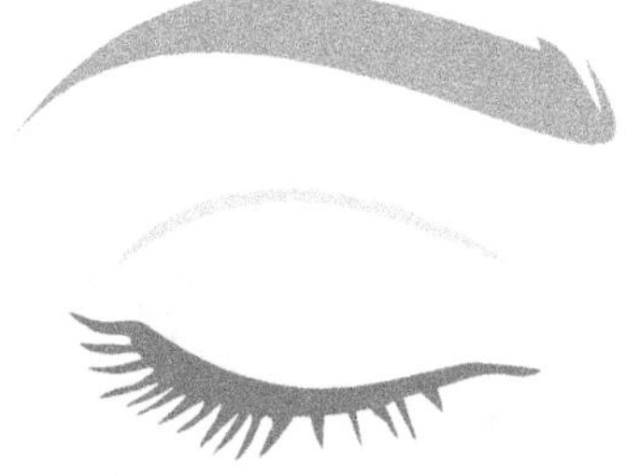
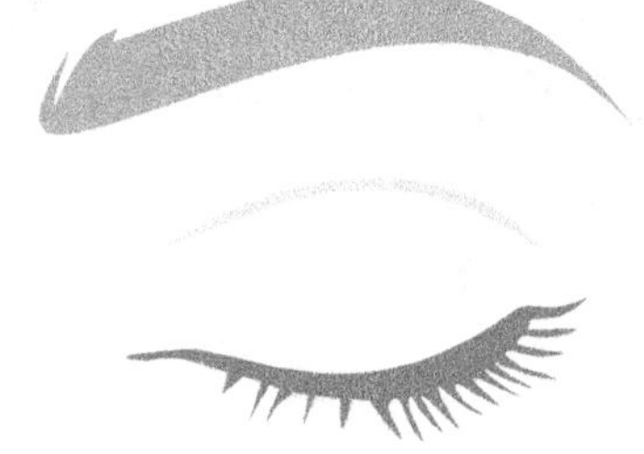
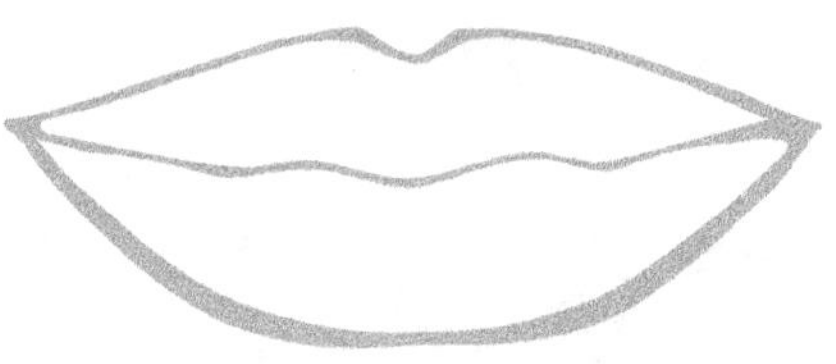

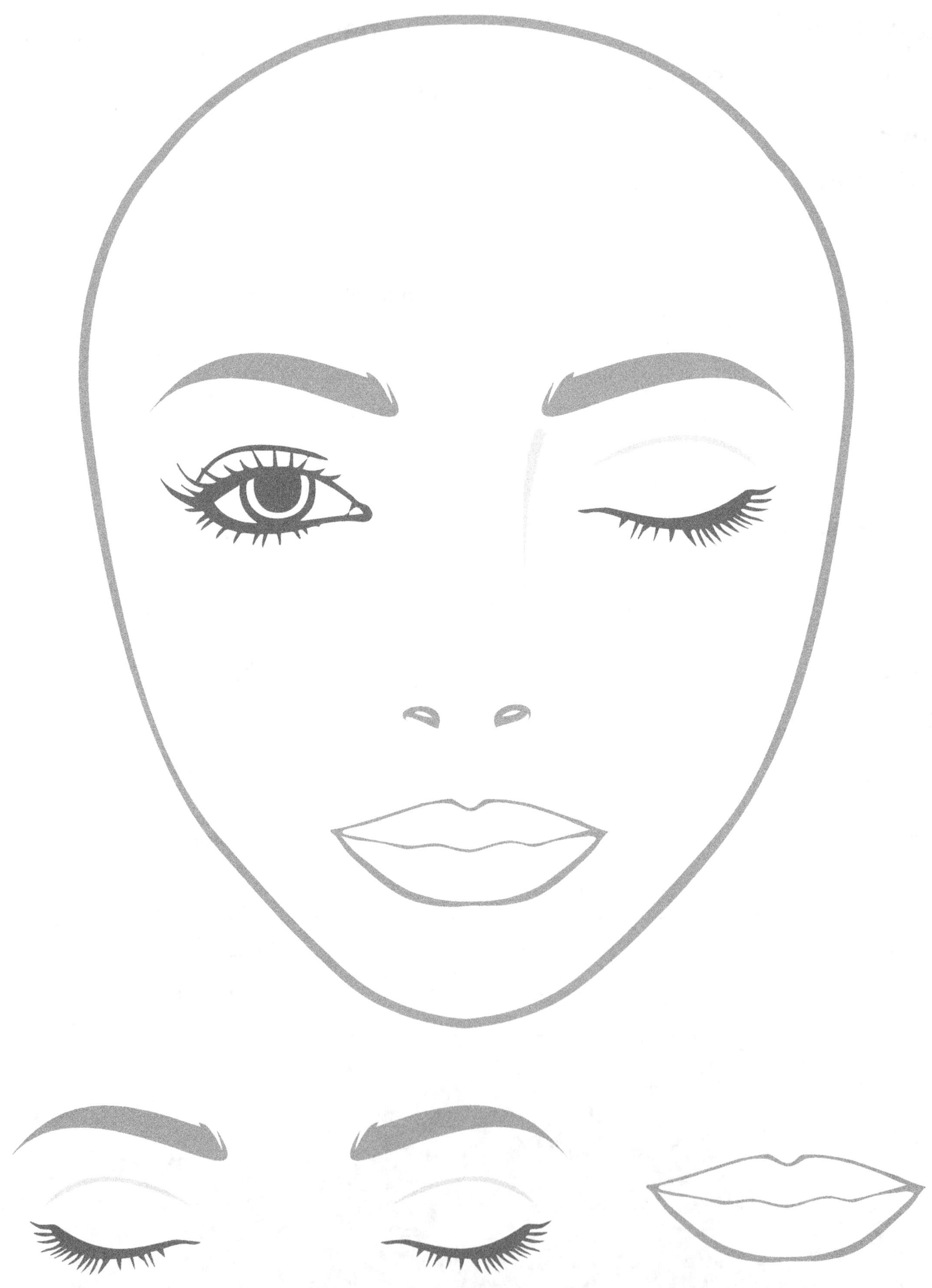

LOOK NAME _______________________   FOR: _______________________

○ Daytime   ○ Evening

FACE

Moisturizer

____

Primer

____

Powder

____

Highlight/Blush

____

Concealer

____

Foundation

____

Contour

____

EYES

Brows	Crease
Eyelid	Mascara
Liner	

LIPS

Liner

Lip Color

Gloss

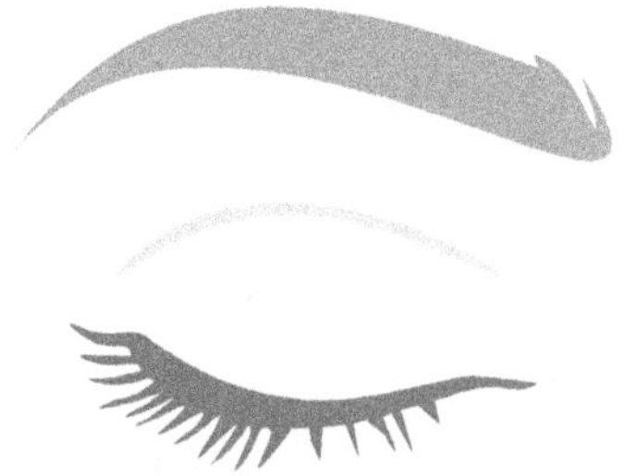
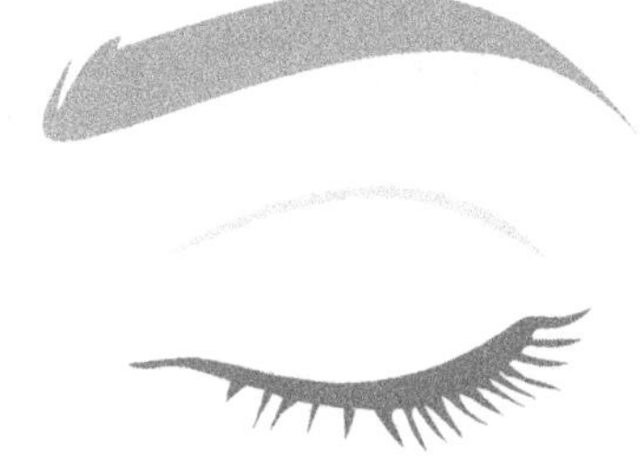
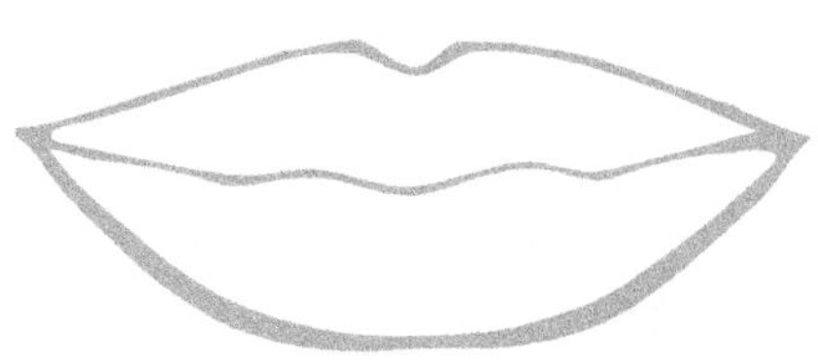

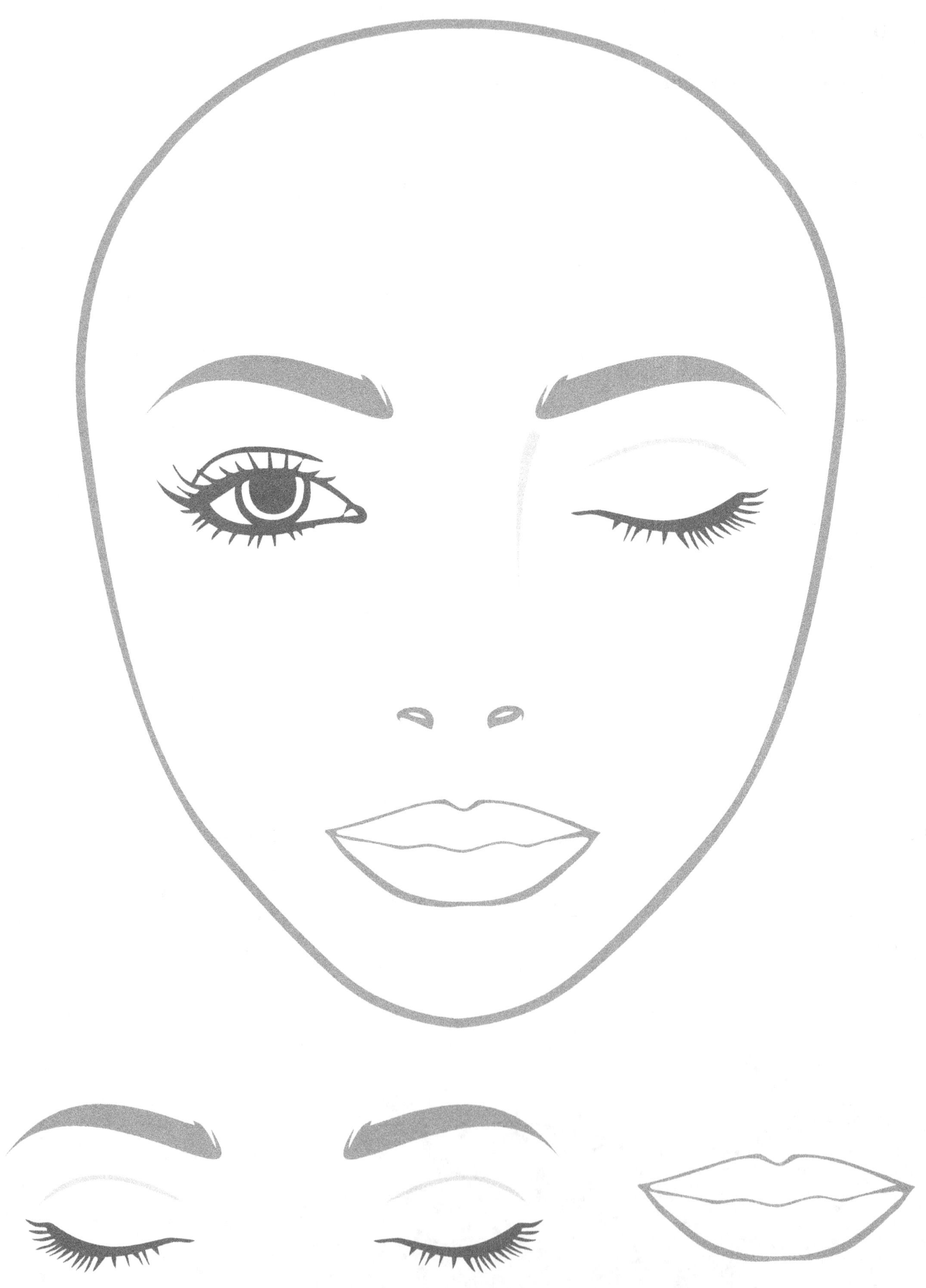

LOOK NAME _______________________   FOR: _______________________

○ Daytime   ○ Evening

FACE

Moisturizer

____

Primer

____

Powder

____

Highlight/Blush

____

Concealer

____

Foundation

____

Contour

____

EYES

Brows	Crease	
Eyelid	Mascara	
Liner		

LIPS

Liner

____

Lip Color

____

Gloss

____

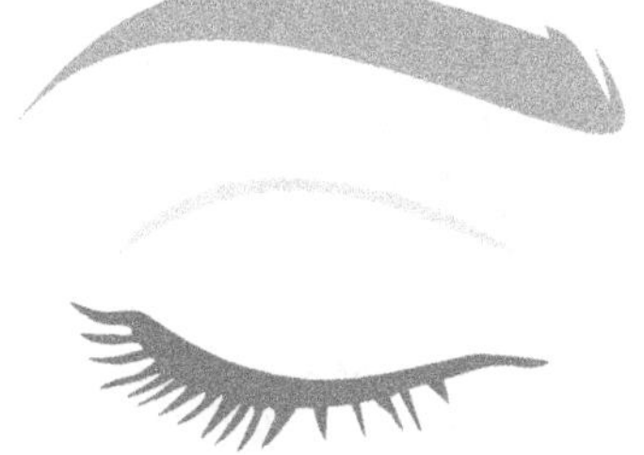
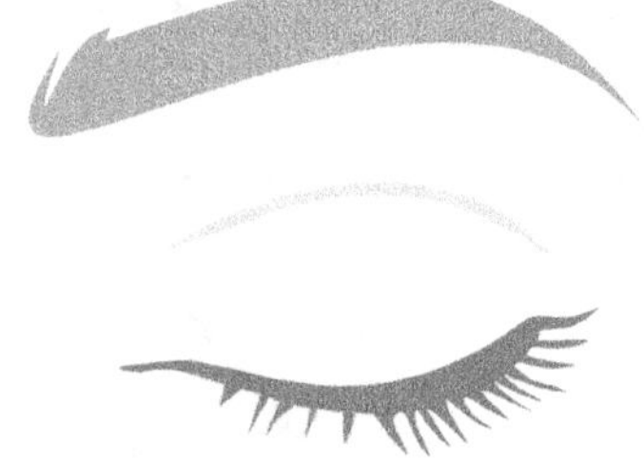
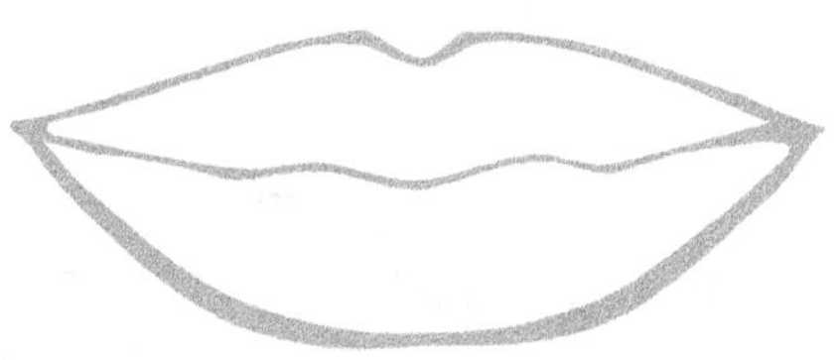

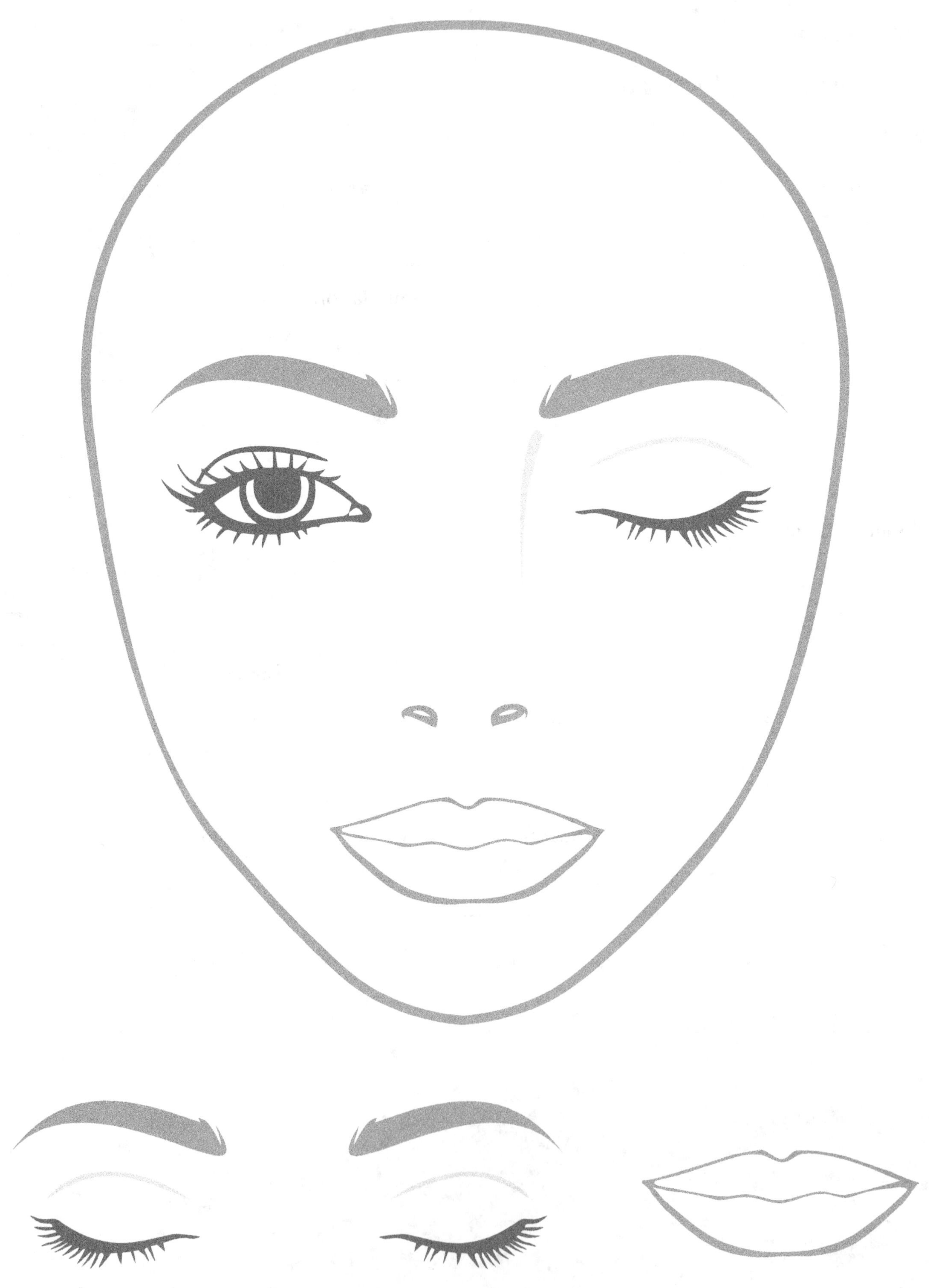

LOOK NAME ______________________   FOR: ______________________

◯ Daytime   ◯ Evening

FACE

Moisturizer

____

Primer

____

Powder

____

Highlight/Blush

____

Concealer

____

Foundation

____

Contour

____

EYES

Brows

____

Eyelid

____

Liner

____

Crease

____

Mascara

____

LIPS

Liner

____

Lip Color

____

Gloss

____

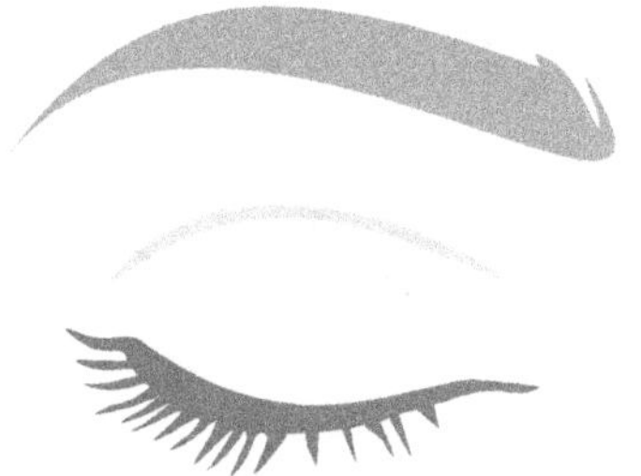
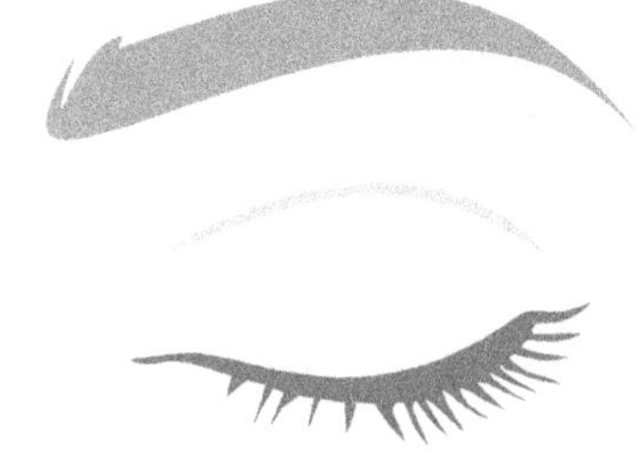
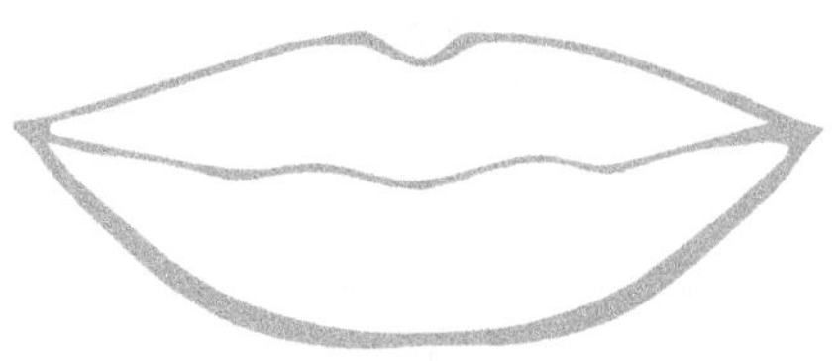

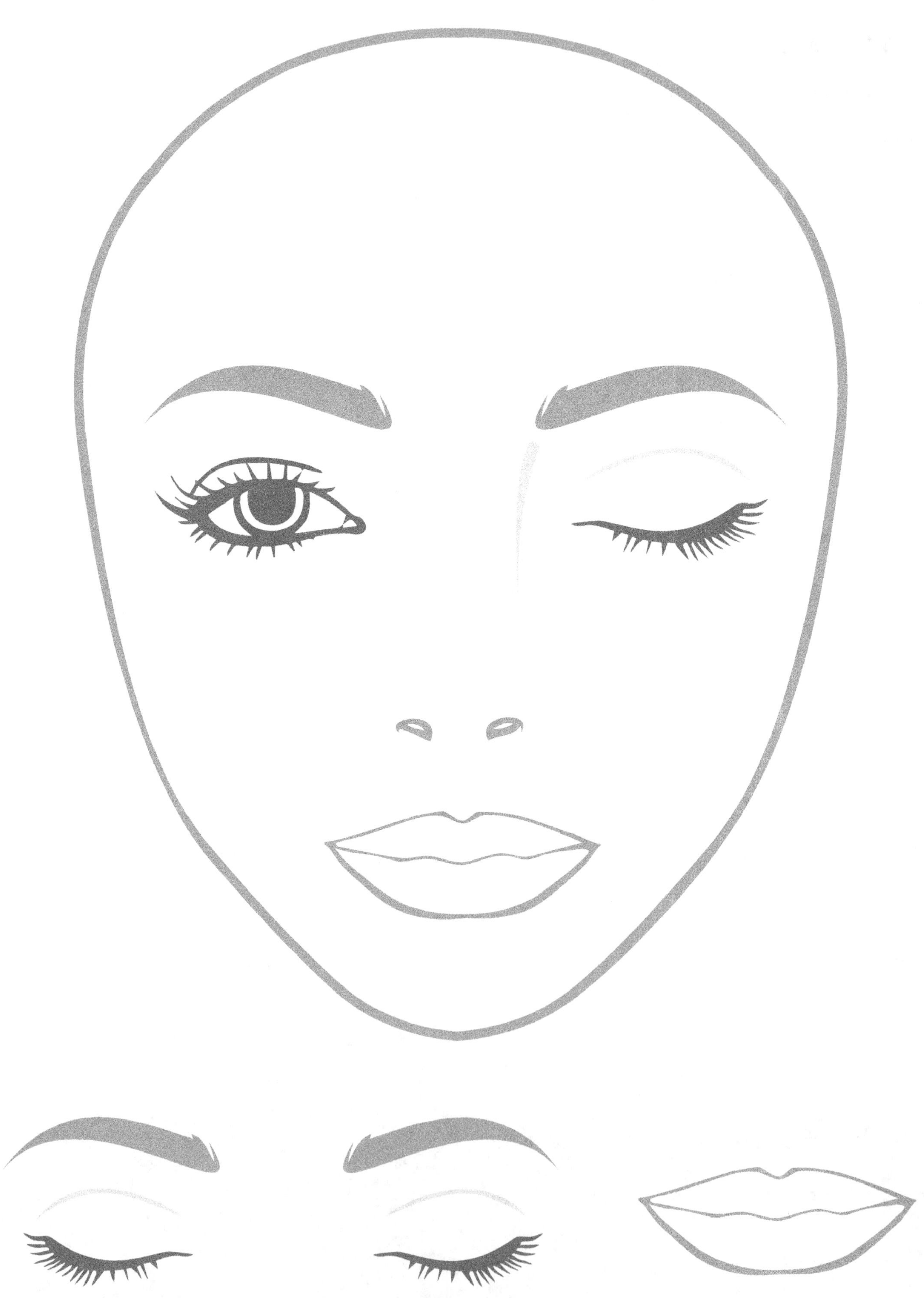

LOOK NAME _______________________   FOR: _______________

◯ Daytime   ◯ Evening

FACE

Moisturizer

____

Primer

____

Powder

____

Highlight/Blush

____

Concealer

____

Foundation

____

Contour

____

EYES

Brows

____

Eyelid

____

Liner

____

Crease

____

Mascara

____

LIPS

Liner

____

Lip Color

____

Gloss

____

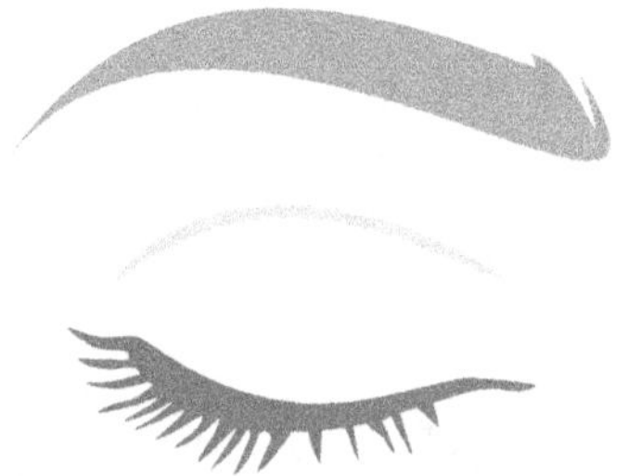

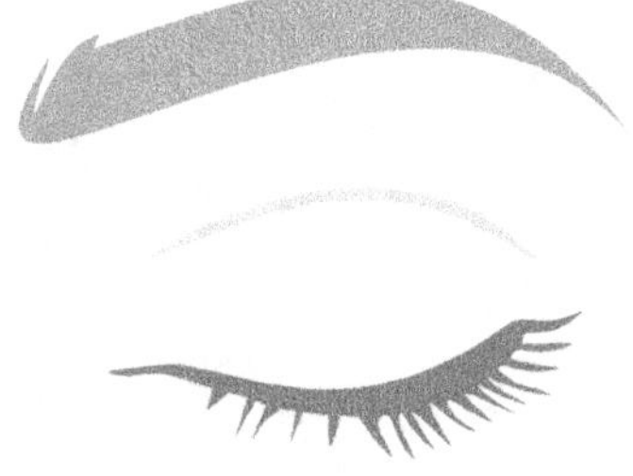

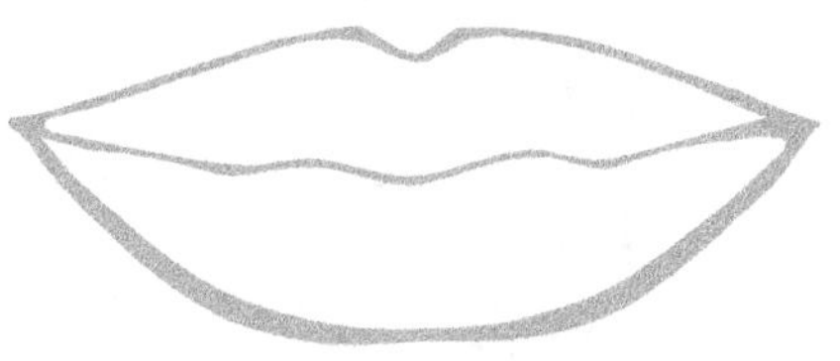

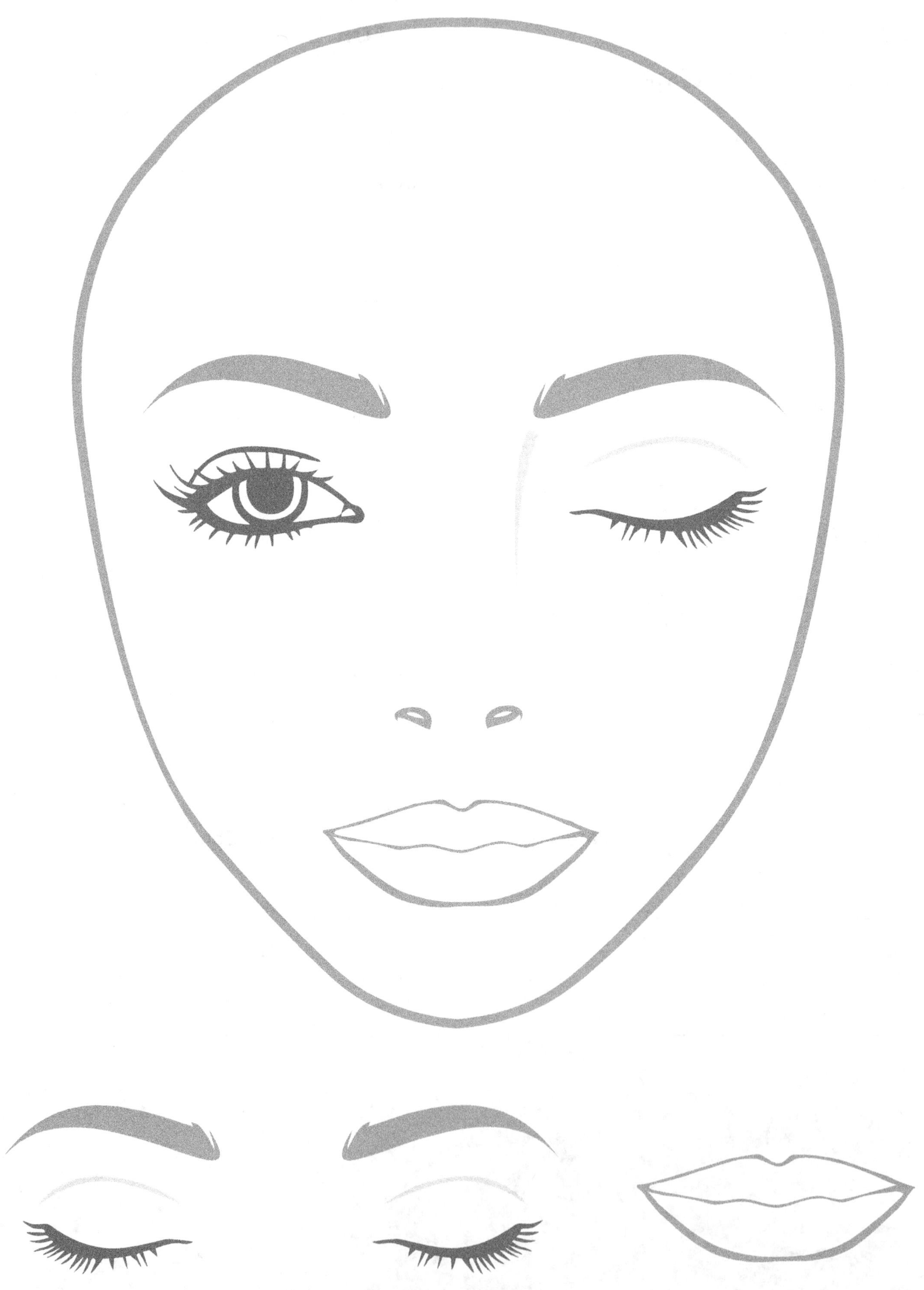

LOOK NAME ________________   FOR: ________________

○ Daytime   ○ Evening

FACE

Moisturizer

____

Primer

____

Powder

____

Highlight/Blush

____

Concealer

____

Foundation

____

Contour

____

EYES

Brows

____

Eyelid

____

Liner

____

Crease

____

Mascara

____

LIPS

Liner

____

Lip Color

____

Gloss

____

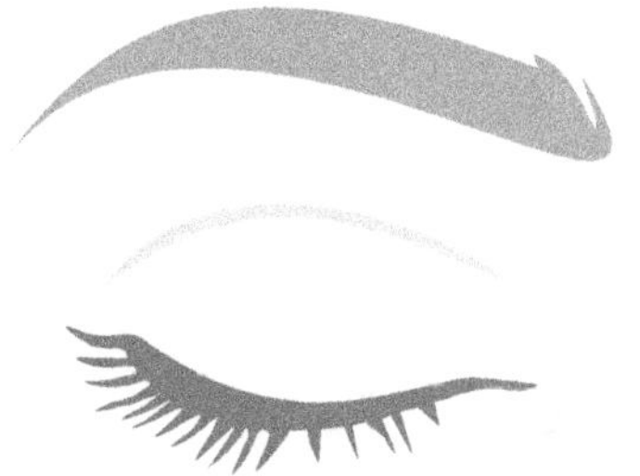
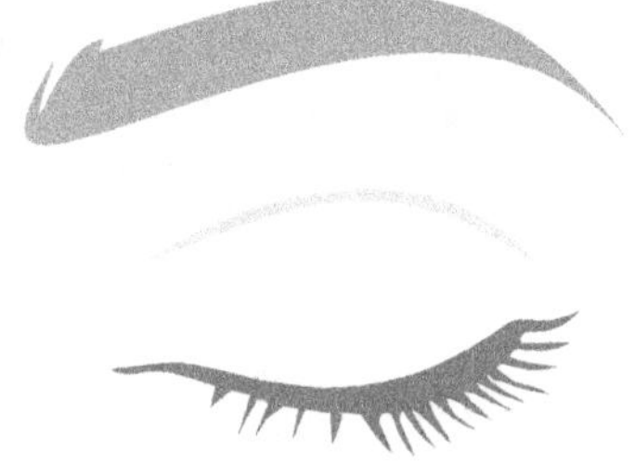
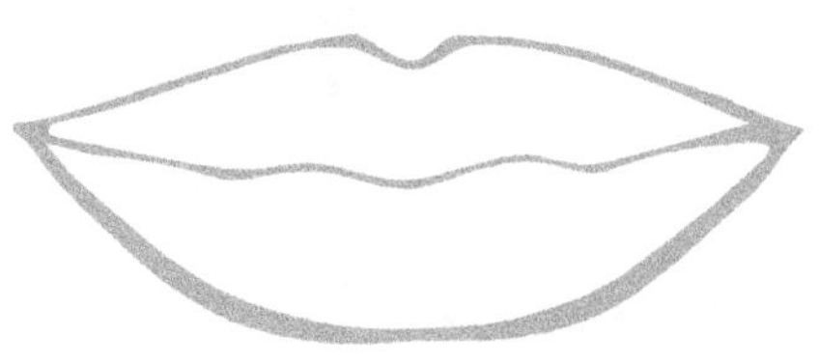

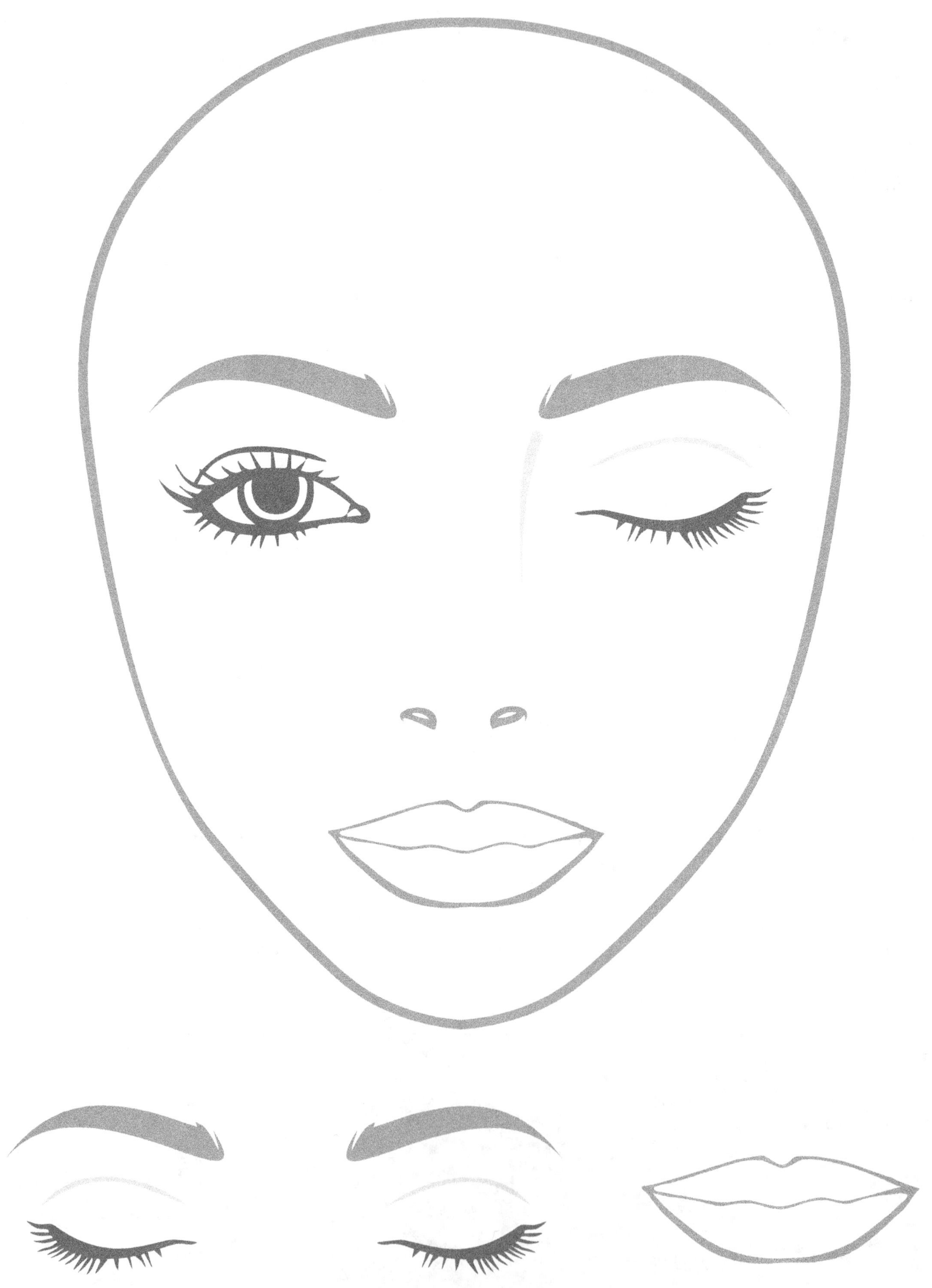

LOOK NAME ________________________   FOR: __________________

◯ Daytime   ◯ Evening

FACE

Moisturizer

____

Primer

____

Powder

____

Highlight/Blush

____

Concealer

____

Foundation

____

Contour

____

EYES

Brows

____

Eyelid

____

Liner

____

Crease

____

Mascara

____

LIPS

Liner

____

Lip Color

____

Gloss

____

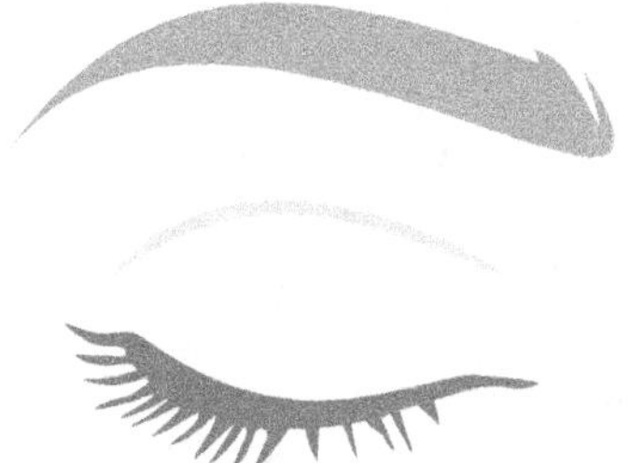
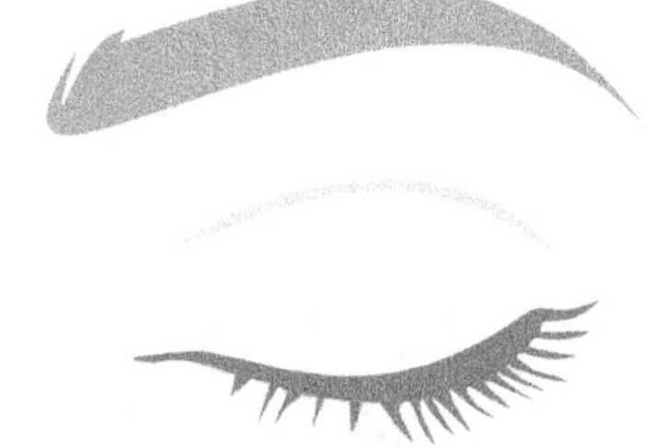
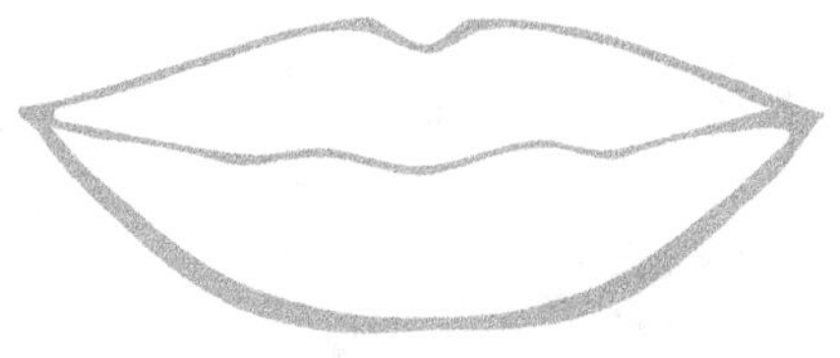

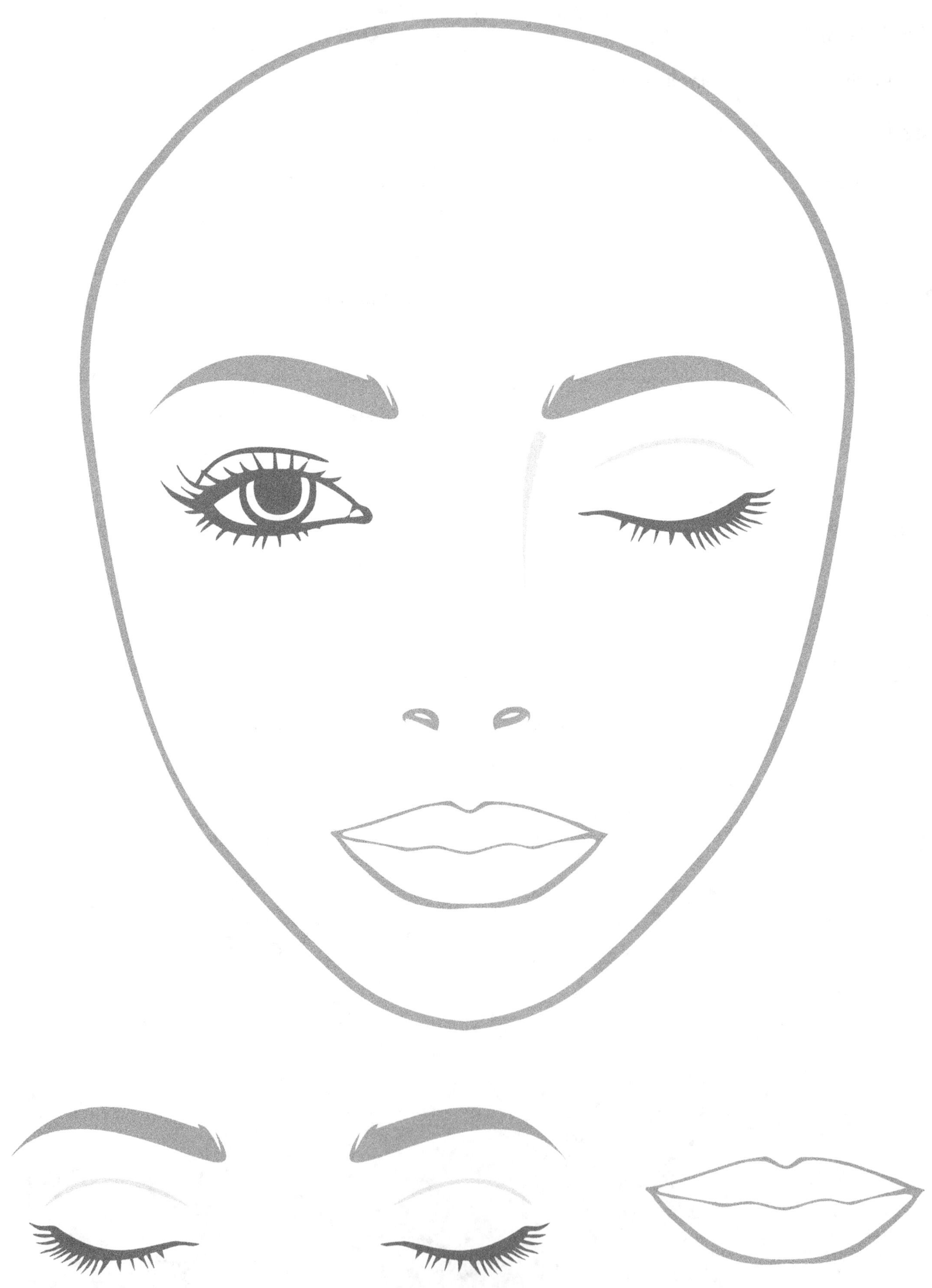

LOOK NAME _______________________   **FOR:** _______________________

◯ Daytime   ◯ Evening

FACE

Moisturizer

Primer

Powder

Highlight/Blush

Concealer

Foundation

Contour

EYES

Brows

Eyelid

Liner

Crease

Mascara

LIPS

Liner

Lip Color

Gloss

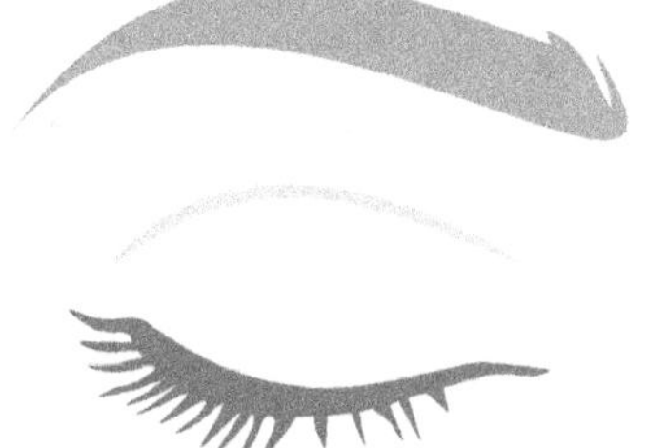
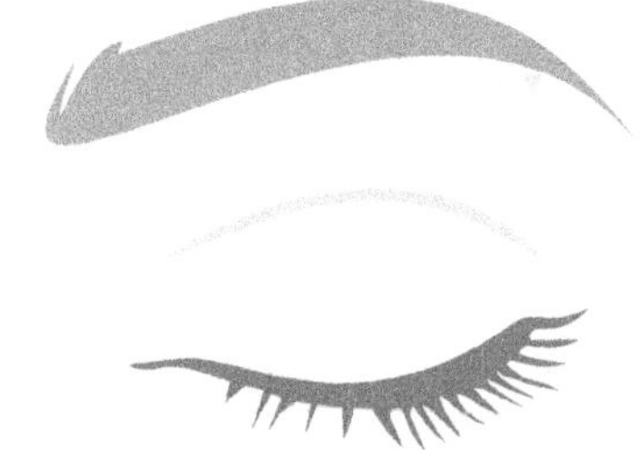
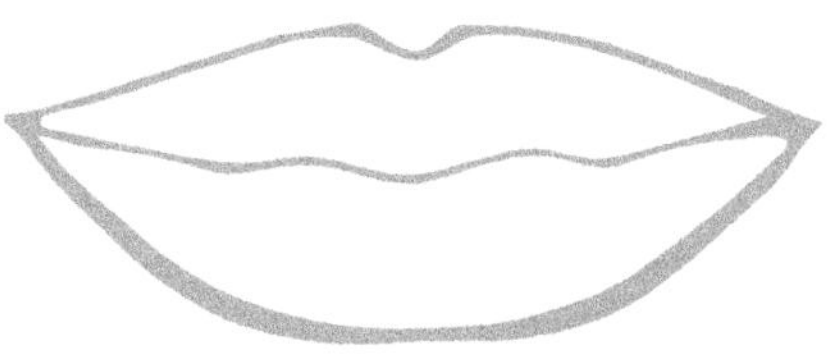

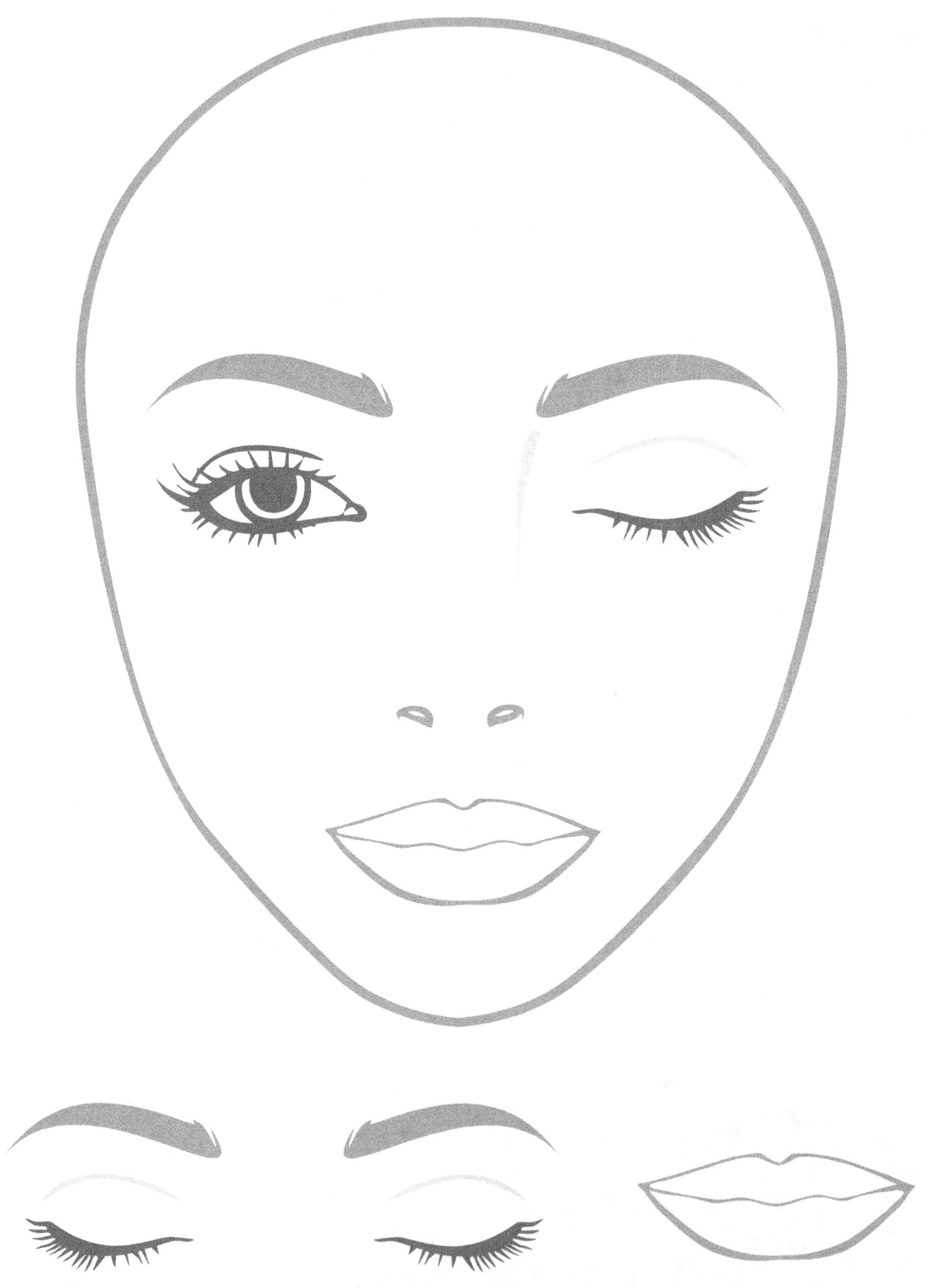

LOOK NAME _________________________   **FOR:** _________________________

◯ Daytime   ◯ Evening

FACE

Moisturizer

____

Primer

____

Powder

____

Highlight/Blush

____

Concealer

____

Foundation

____

Contour

____

EYES

Brows

____

Eyelid

____

Liner

____

Crease

____

Mascara

____

LIPS

Liner

____

Lip Color

____

Gloss

____

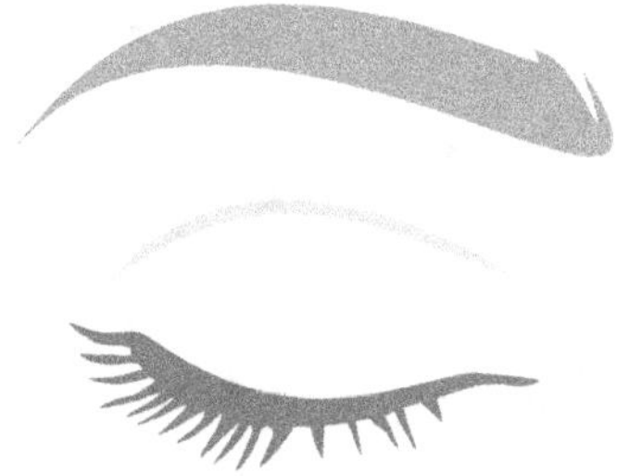
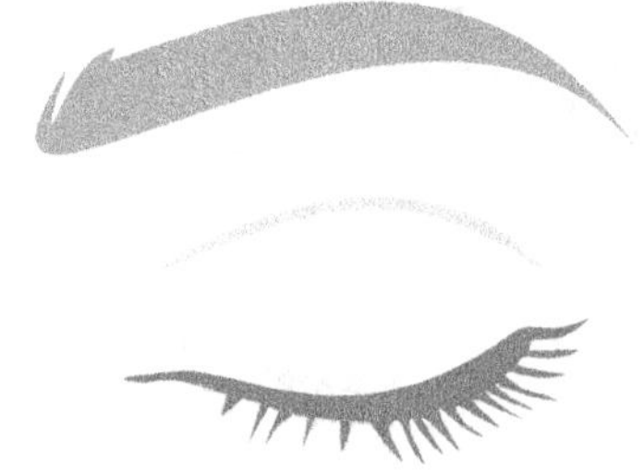
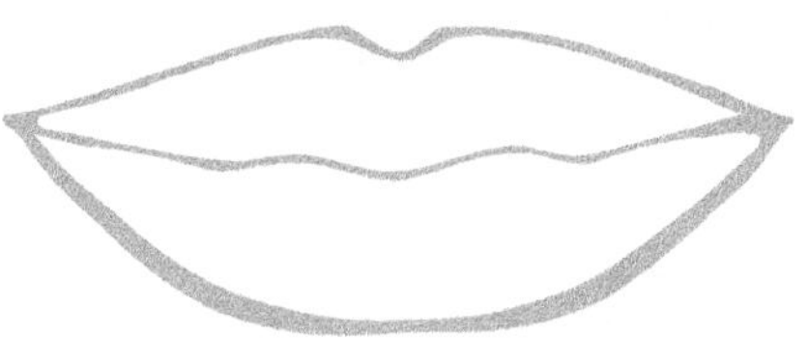

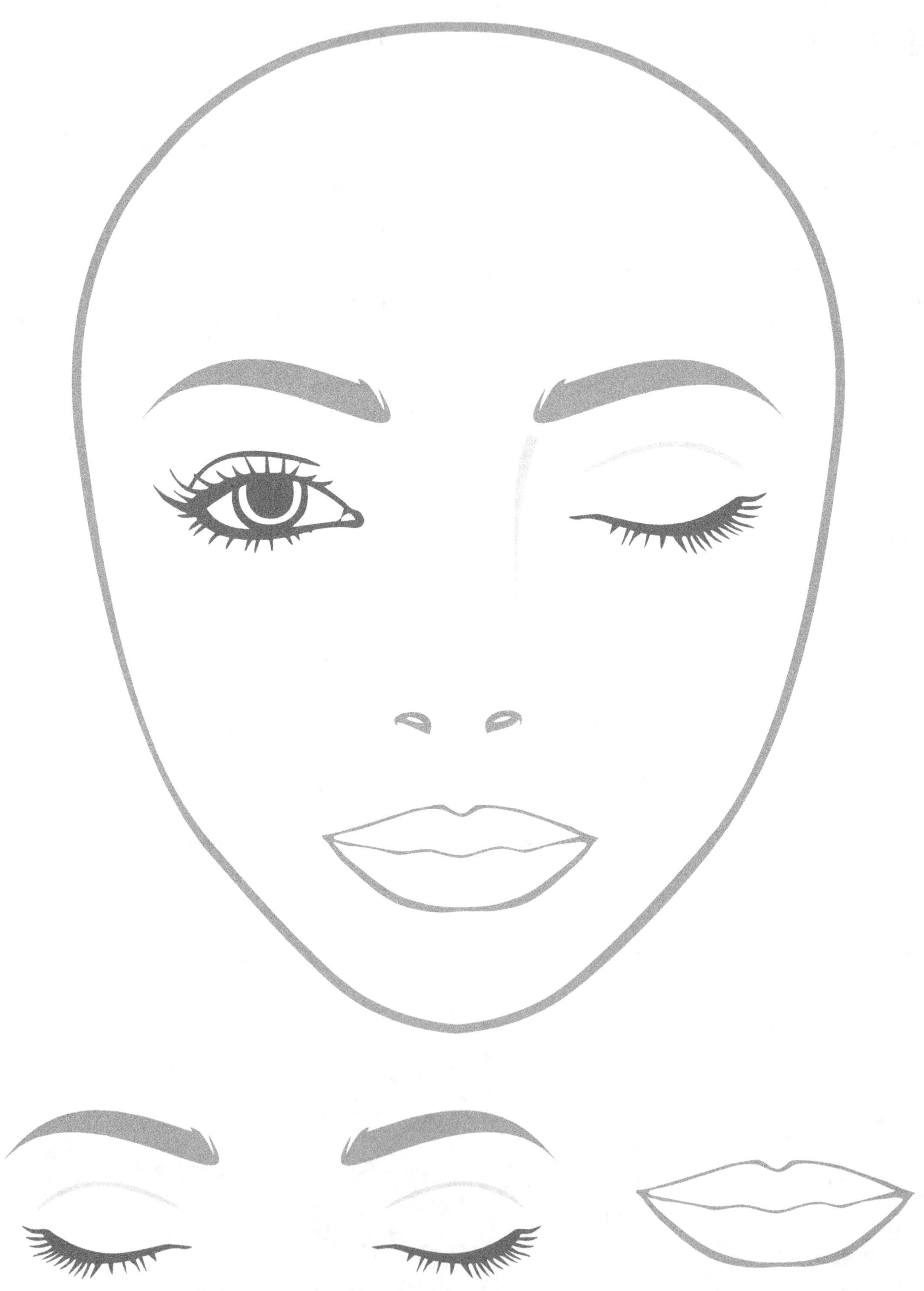

LOOK NAME ________________   FOR: ________________

◯ Daytime   ◯ Evening

FACE

Moisturizer

Primer

Powder

Highlight/Blush

Concealer

Foundation

Contour

EYES

Brows

Eyelid

Liner

Crease

Mascara

LIPS

Liner

Lip Color

Gloss

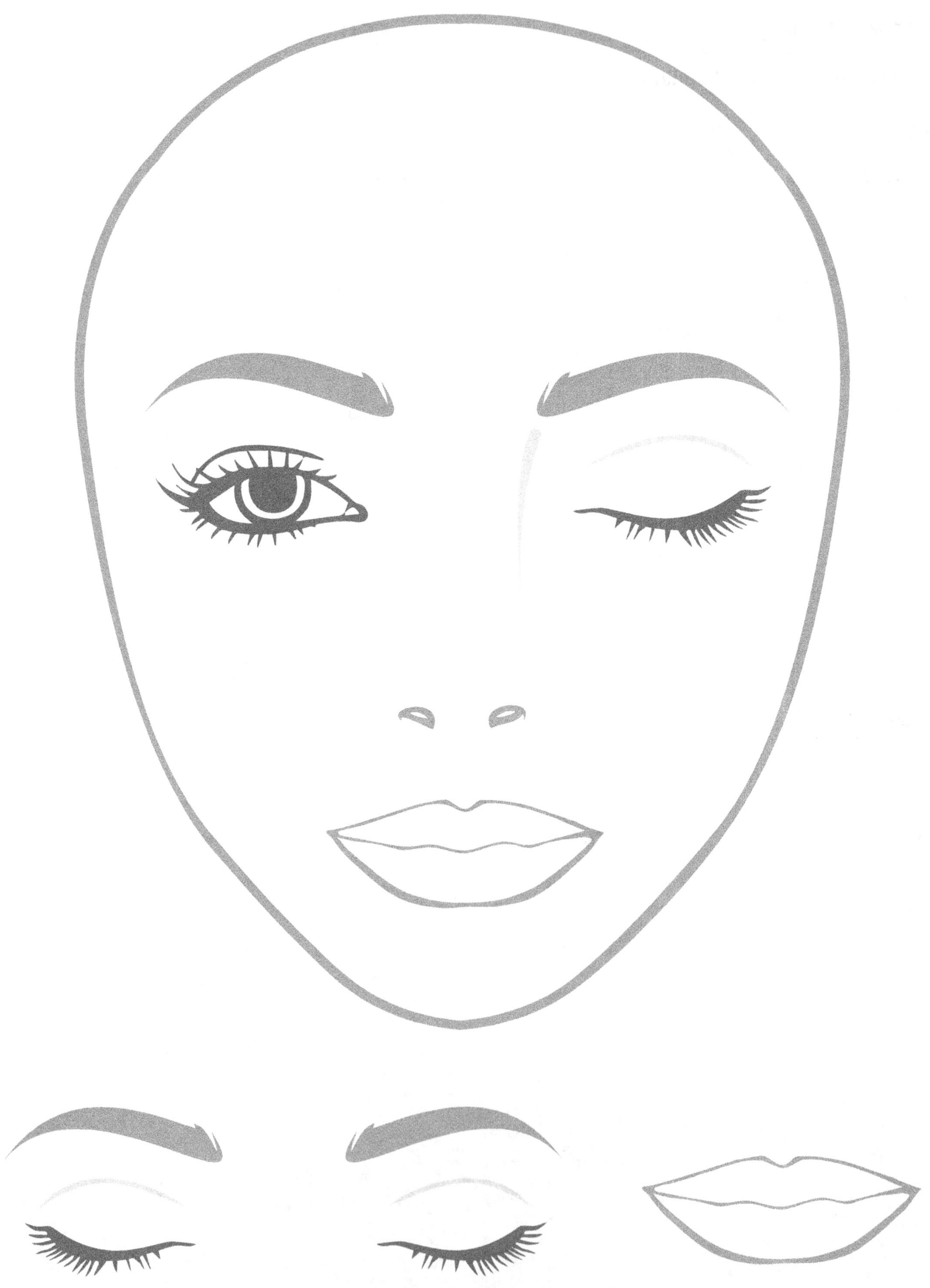

LOOK NAME ______________________   **FOR:** ______________________

◯ Daytime   ◯ Evening

FACE

Moisturizer

____

Primer

____

Powder

____

Highlight/Blush

____

Concealer

____

Foundation

____

Contour

____

EYES

Brows

____

Eyelid

____

Liner

____

Crease

____

Mascara

____

LIPS

Liner

____

Lip Color

____

Gloss

____

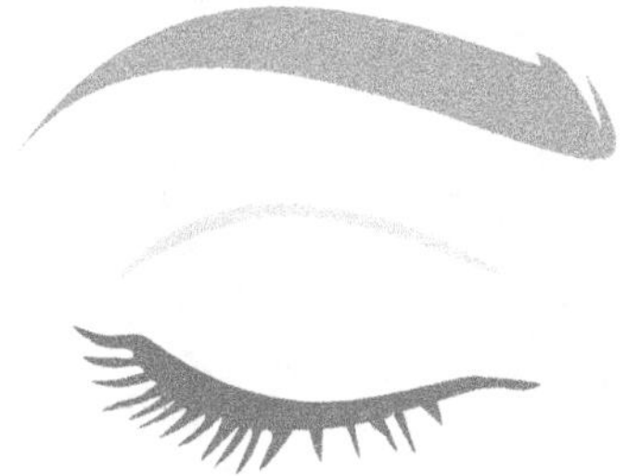
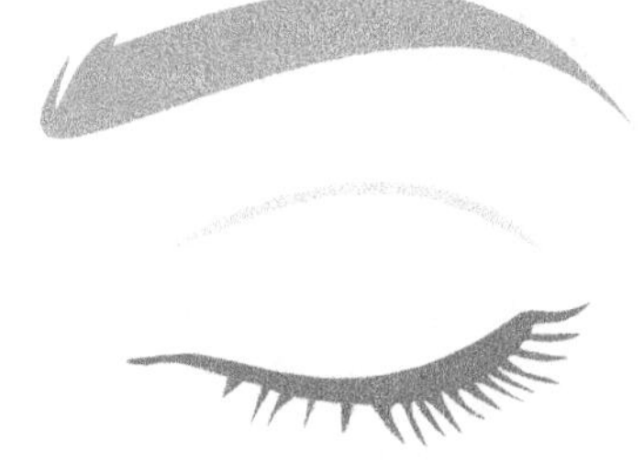
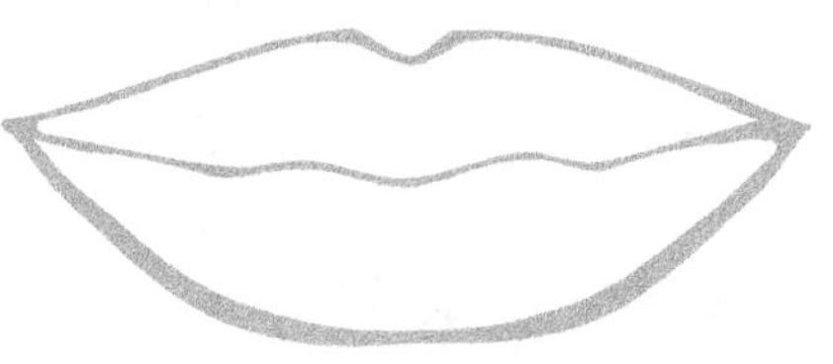

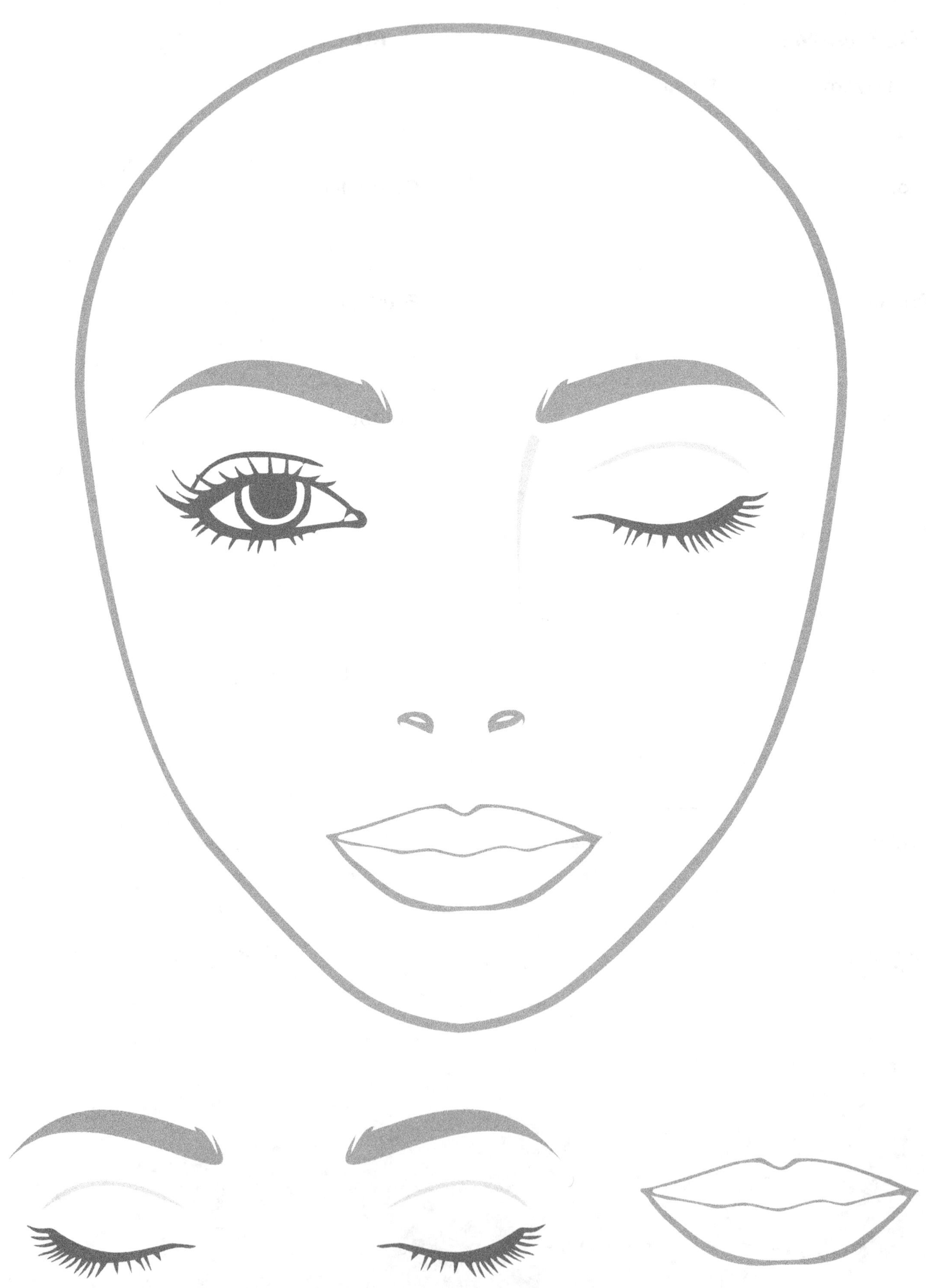

LOOK NAME _______________________   **FOR:** _______________________

◯ Daytime   ◯ Evening

FACE

Moisturizer

____

Primer

____

Powder

____

Highlight/Blush

____

Concealer

____

Foundation

____

Contour

____

EYES

Brows	Crease

Eyelid

Mascara

Liner

LIPS

Liner

Lip Color

Gloss

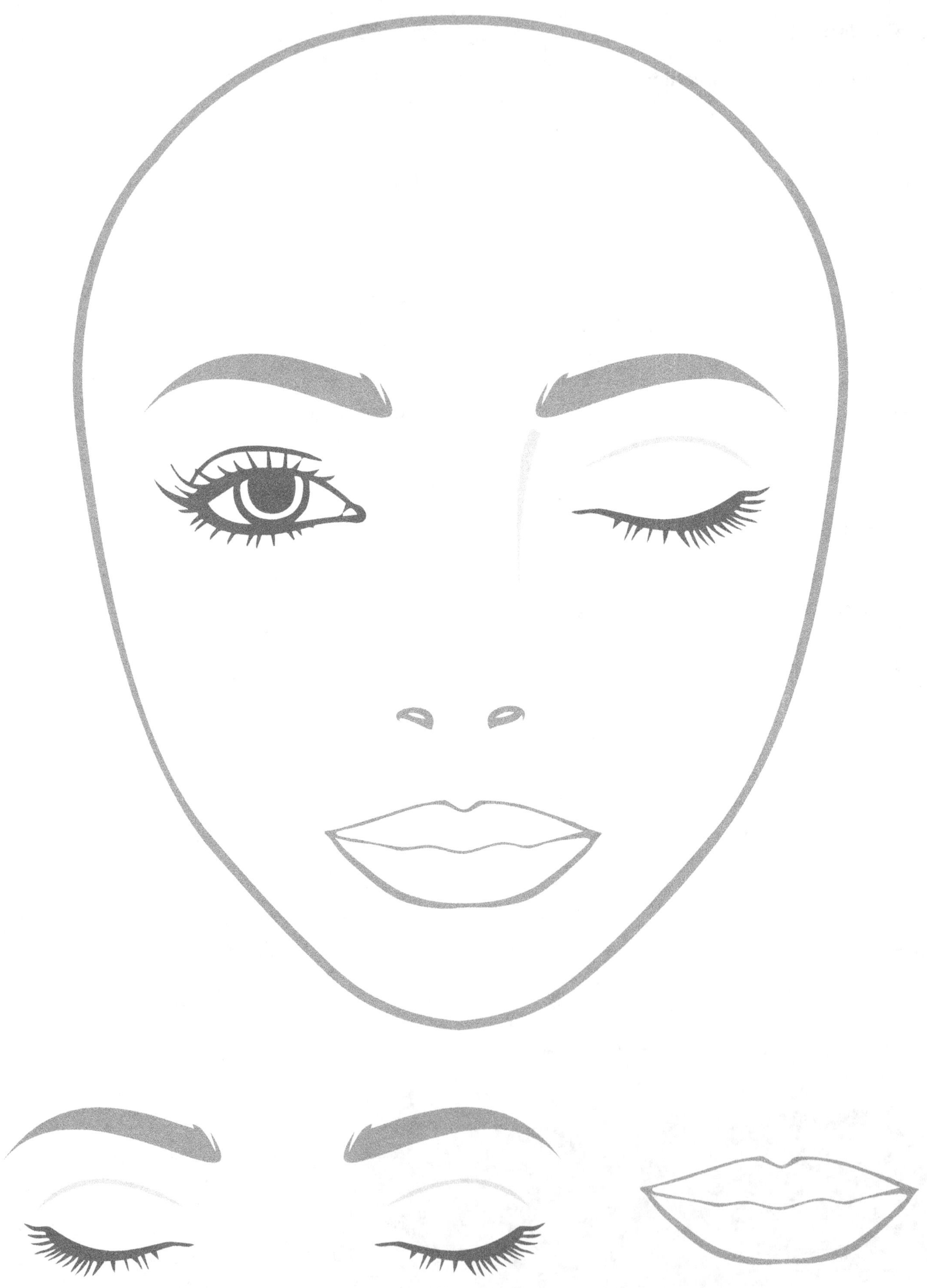

LOOK NAME _______________________   **FOR:** _______________________

◯ Daytime   ◯ Evening

FACE

Moisturizer

____

Primer

____

Powder

____

Highlight/Blush

____

Concealer

____

Foundation

____

Contour

____

EYES

Brows

____

Eyelid

____

Liner

____

Crease

____

Mascara

____

LIPS

Liner

____

Lip Color

____

Gloss

____

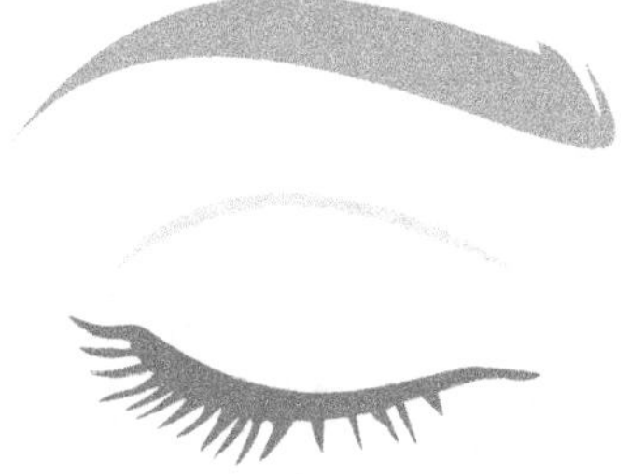

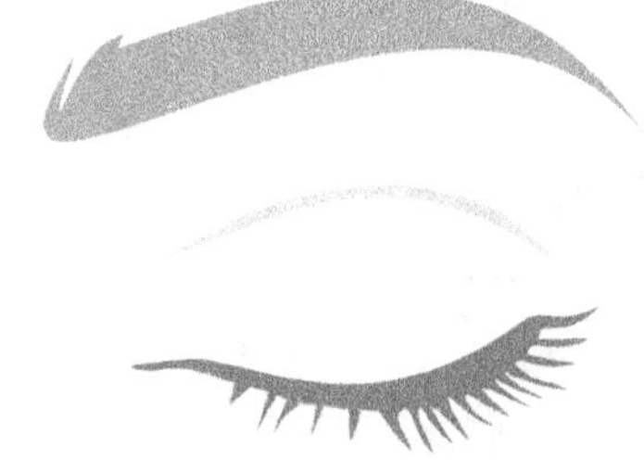

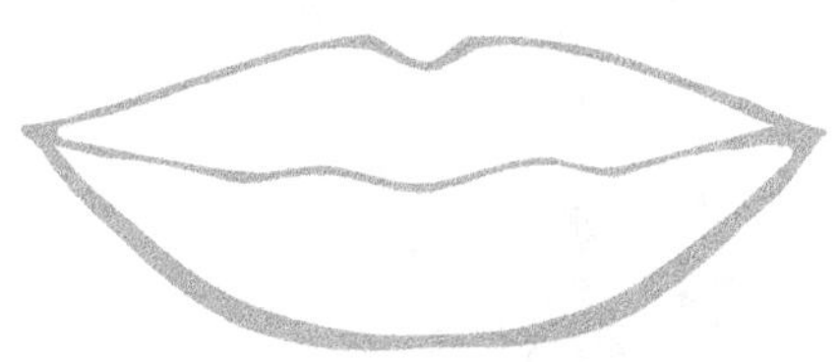

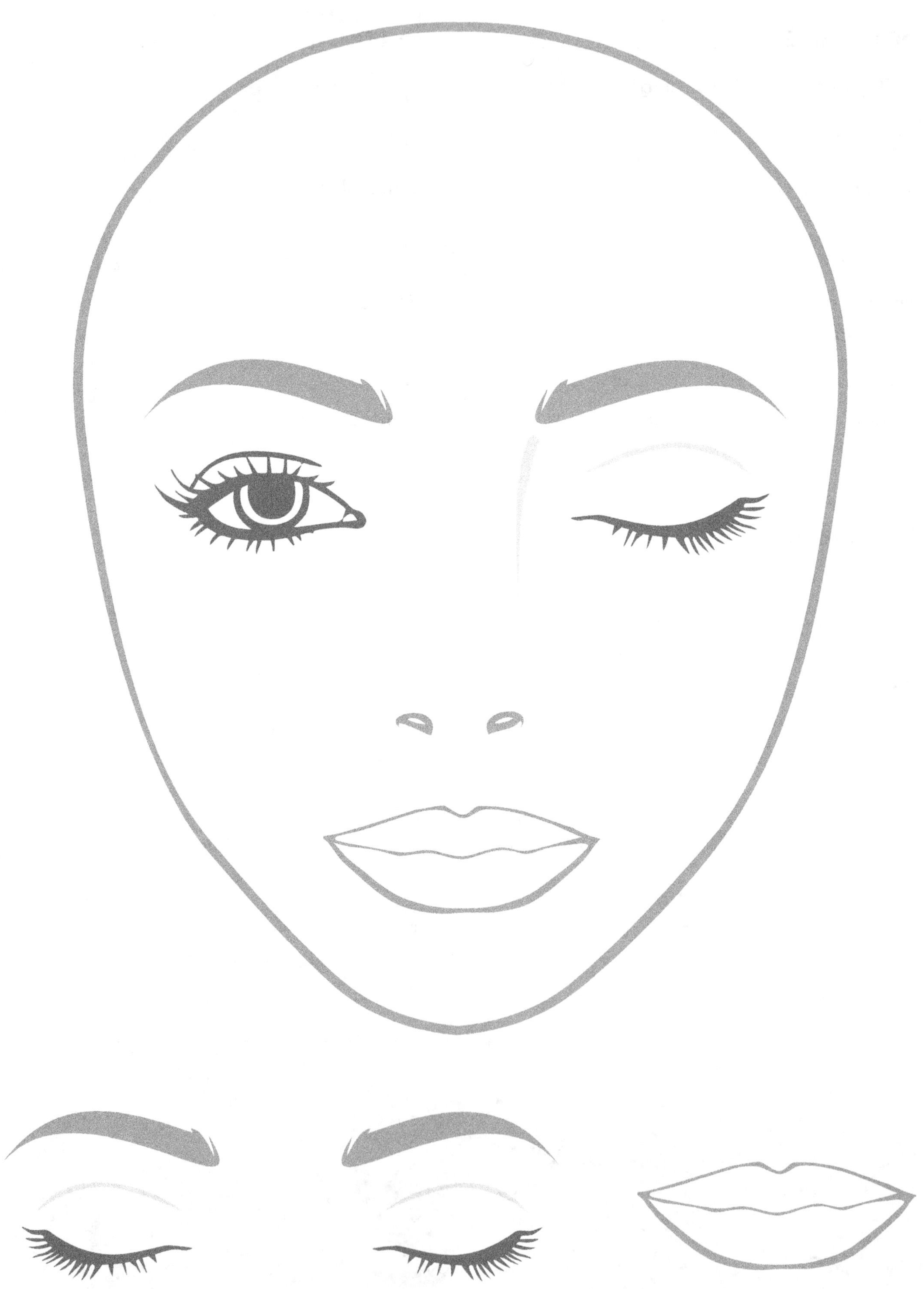

LOOK NAME _______________   FOR: _______________

◯ Daytime   ◯ Evening

FACE

Moisturizer

____

Primer

____

Powder

____

Highlight/Blush

____

Concealer

____

Foundation

____

Contour

____

EYES

Brows

____

Eyelid

____

Liner

____

Crease

____

Mascara

____

LIPS

Liner

____

Lip Color

____

Gloss

____

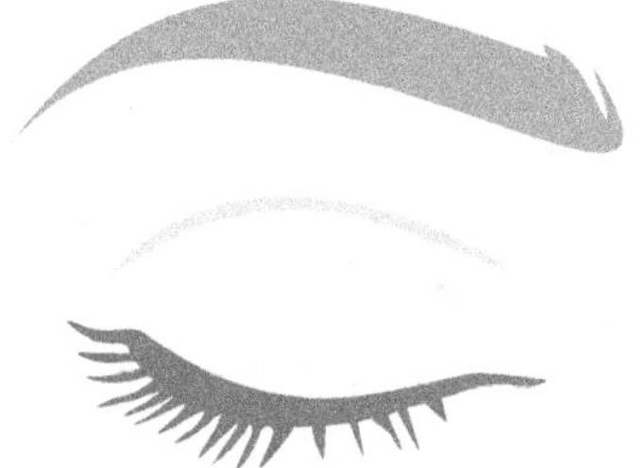

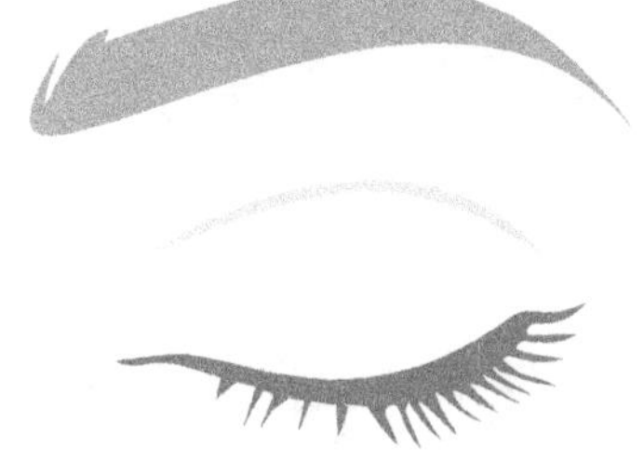

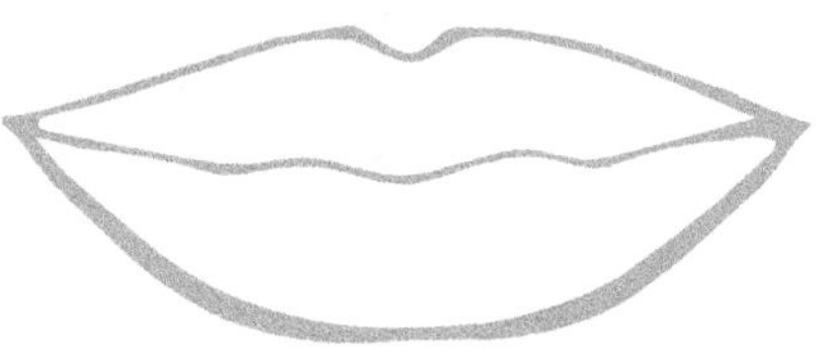

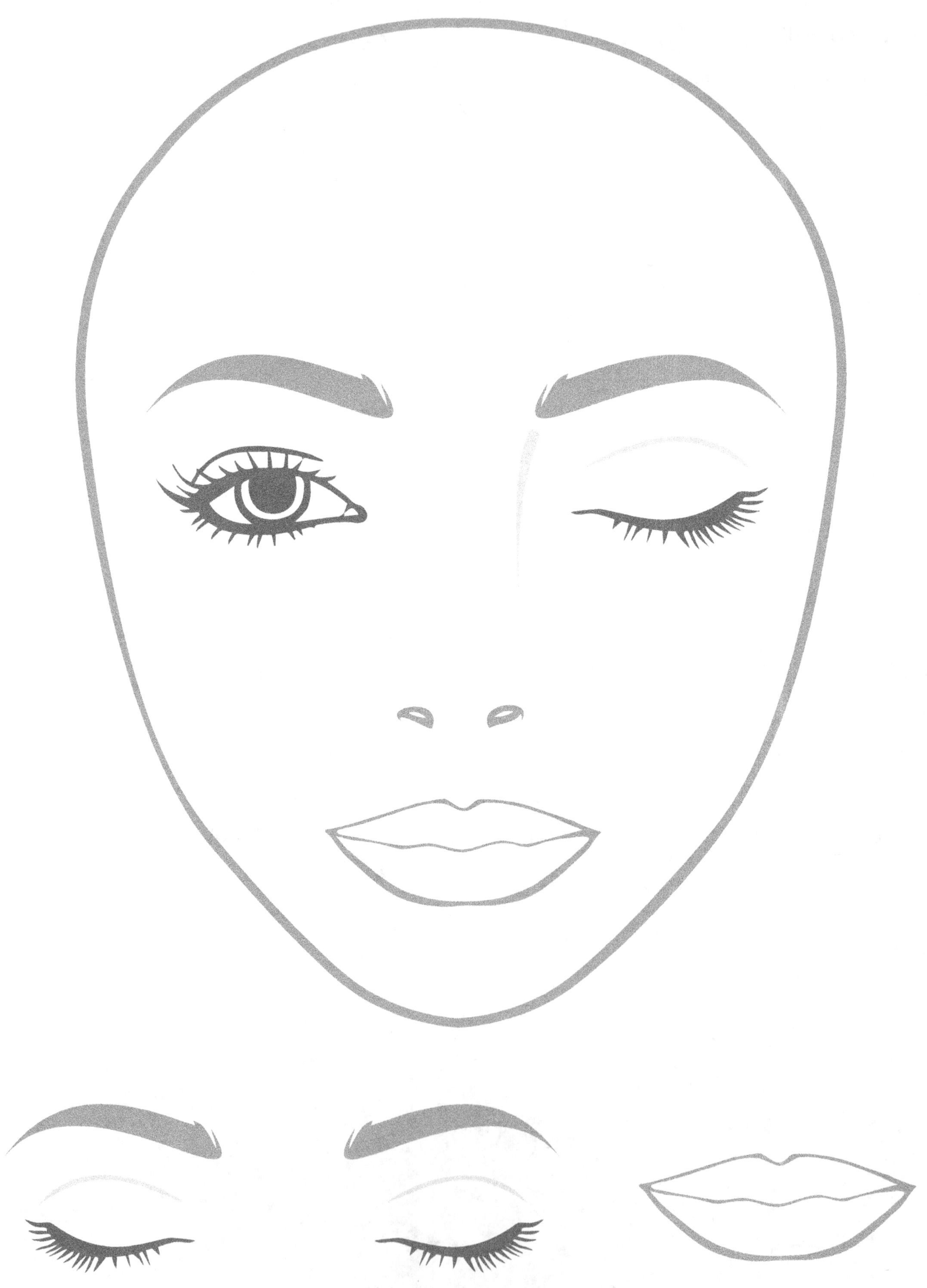

LOOK NAME _______________________________   **FOR:** _______________________________

◯ Daytime   ◯ Evening

FACE

Moisturizer   Concealer

_______________________________   _______________________________

Primer   Foundation

_______________________________   _______________________________

Powder   Contour

_______________________________   _______________________________

Highlight/Blush

____

EYES   ## LIPS

Brows   Crease   Liner

______________   ______________   ______________

Eyelid   Mascara   Lip Color

______________   ______________   ______________

Liner   Gloss

______________   ______________   ______________

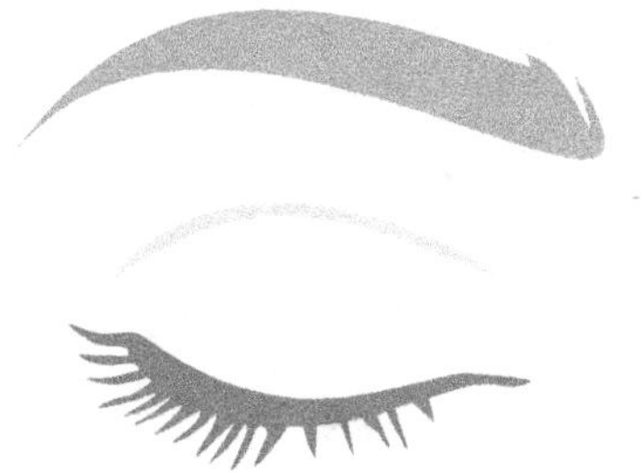 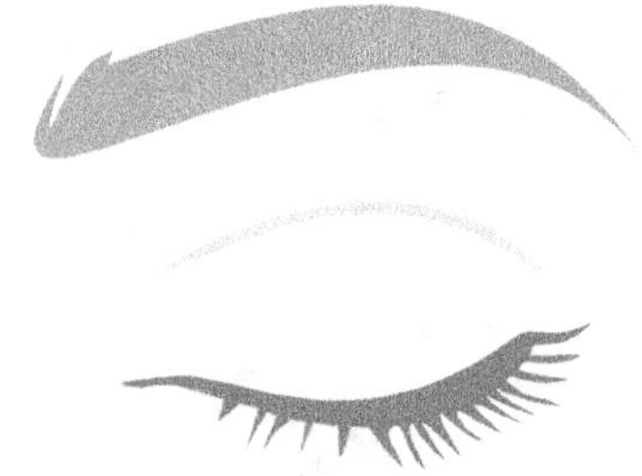 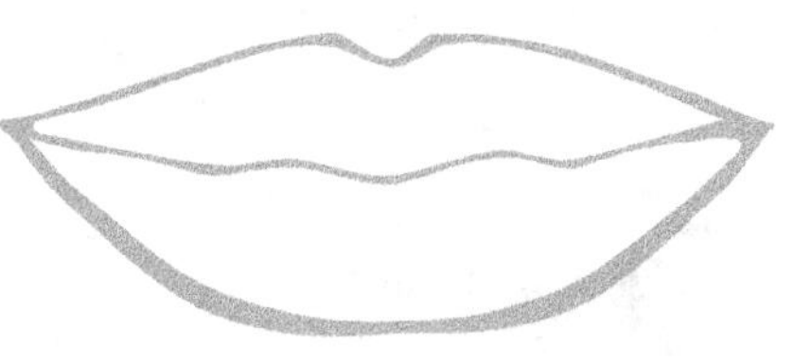

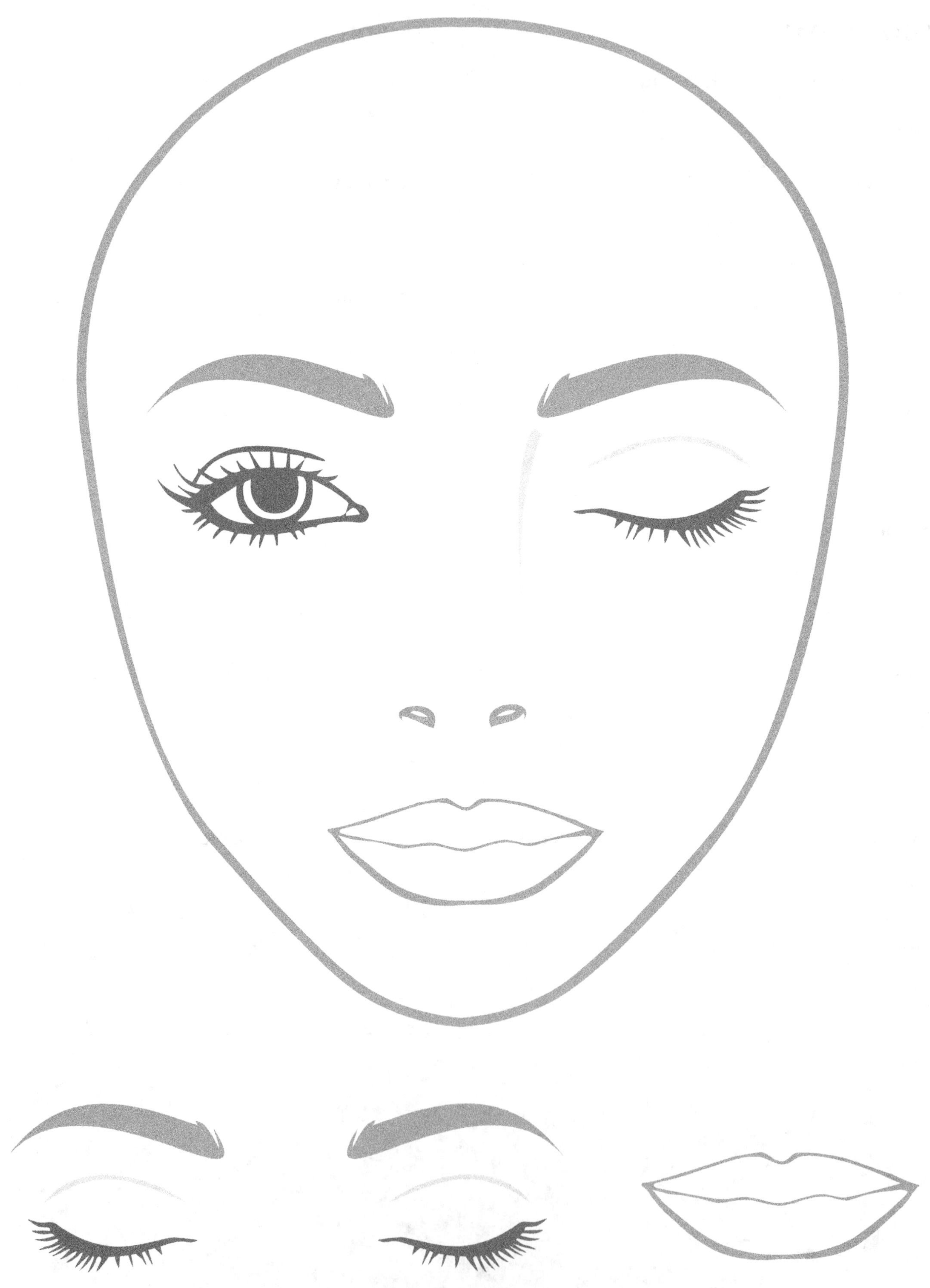

LOOK NAME ______________________ FOR: ______________________

◯ Daytime   ◯ Evening

FACE

Moisturizer

Primer

Powder

Highlight/Blush

Concealer

Foundation

Contour

EYES

Brows

Eyelid

Liner

Crease

Mascara

LIPS

Liner

Lip Color

Gloss

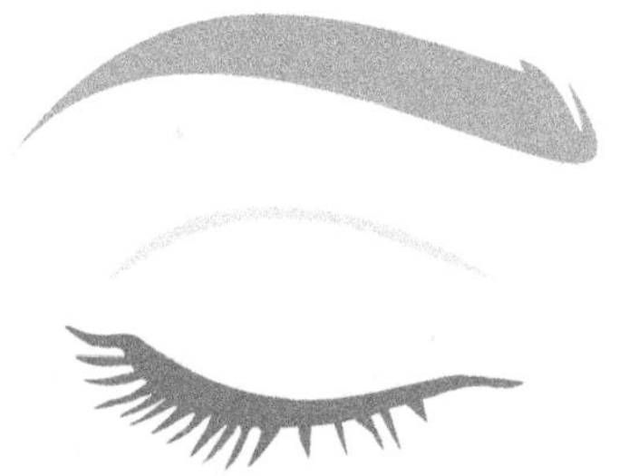

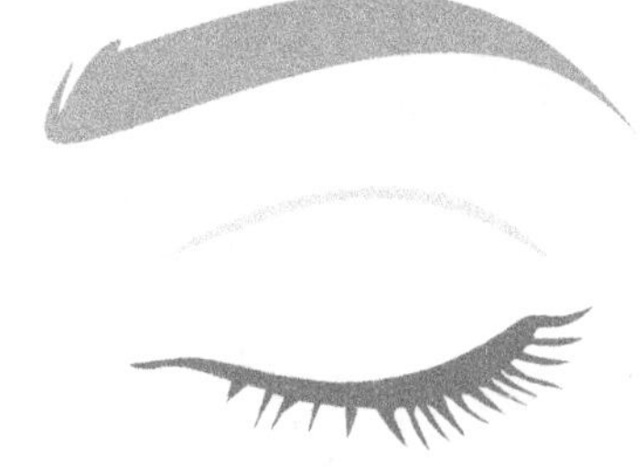

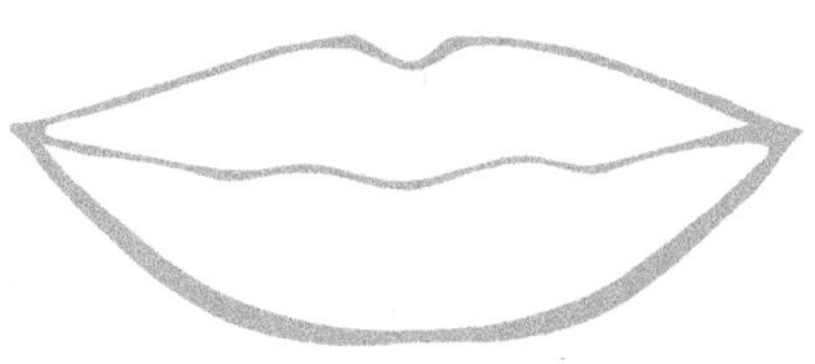

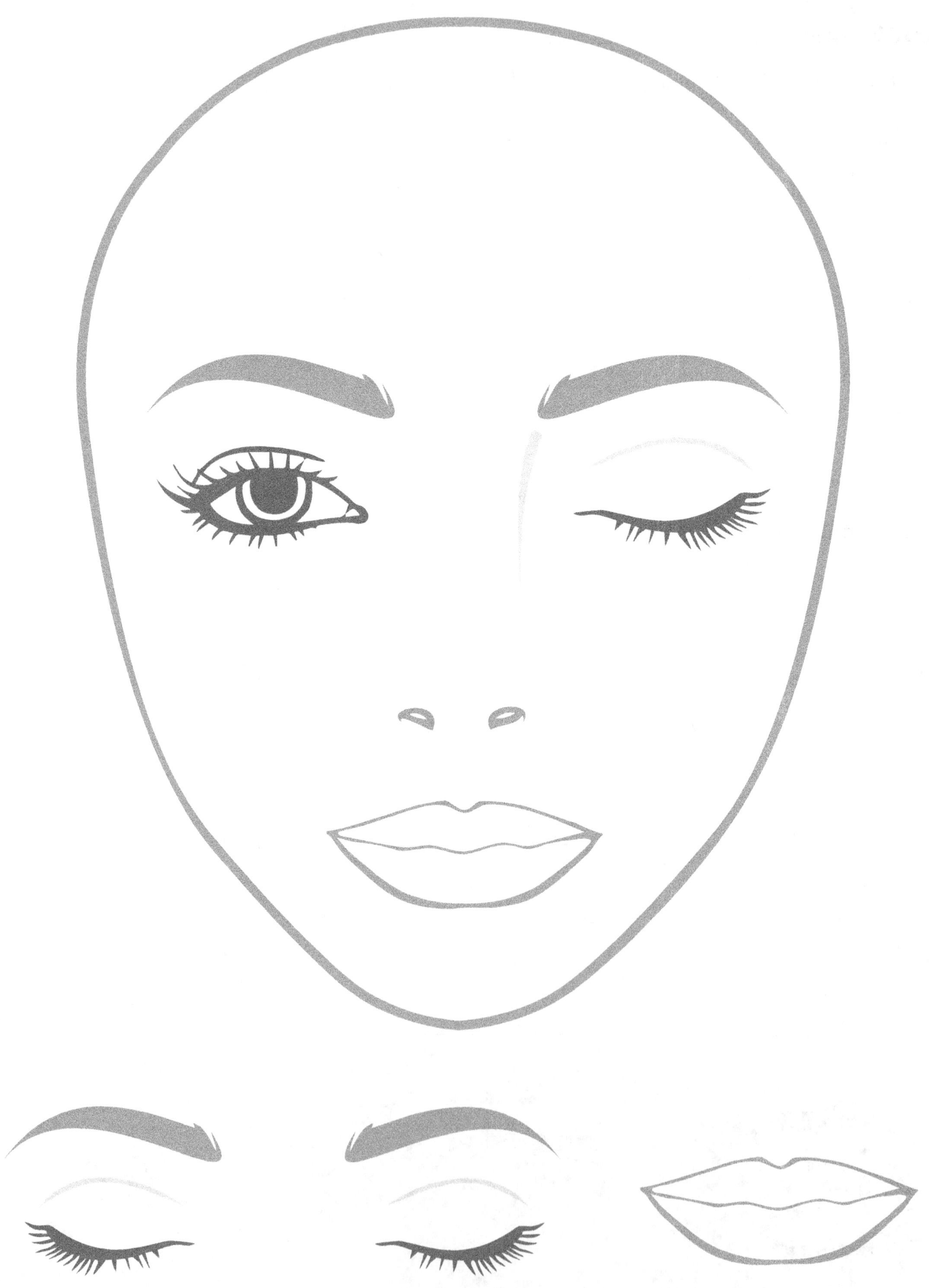

LOOK NAME ________________________ **FOR:** ________________________

◯ Daytime   ◯ Evening

FACE

Moisturizer

Primer

Powder

Highlight/Blush

Concealer

Foundation

Contour

EYES

Brows

Eyelid

Liner

Crease

Mascara

LIPS

Liner

Lip Color

Gloss

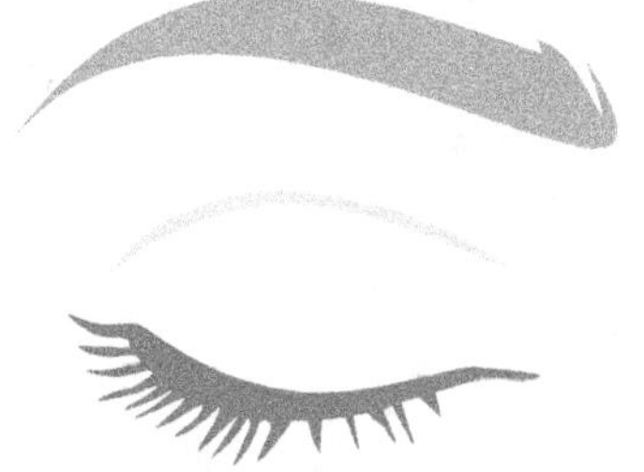

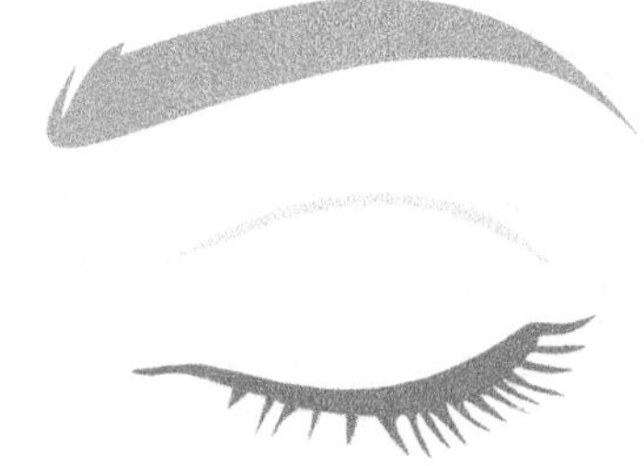

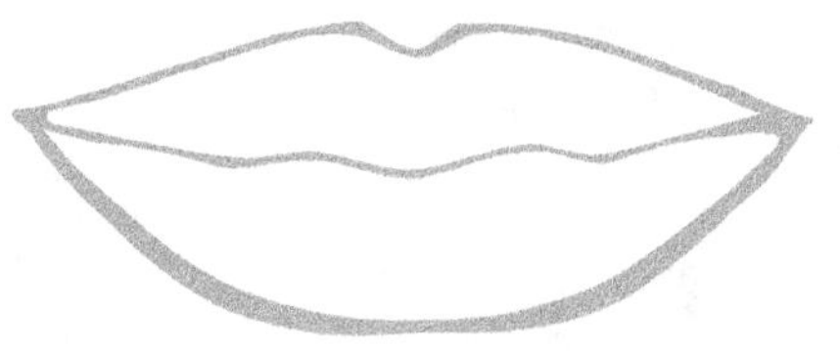

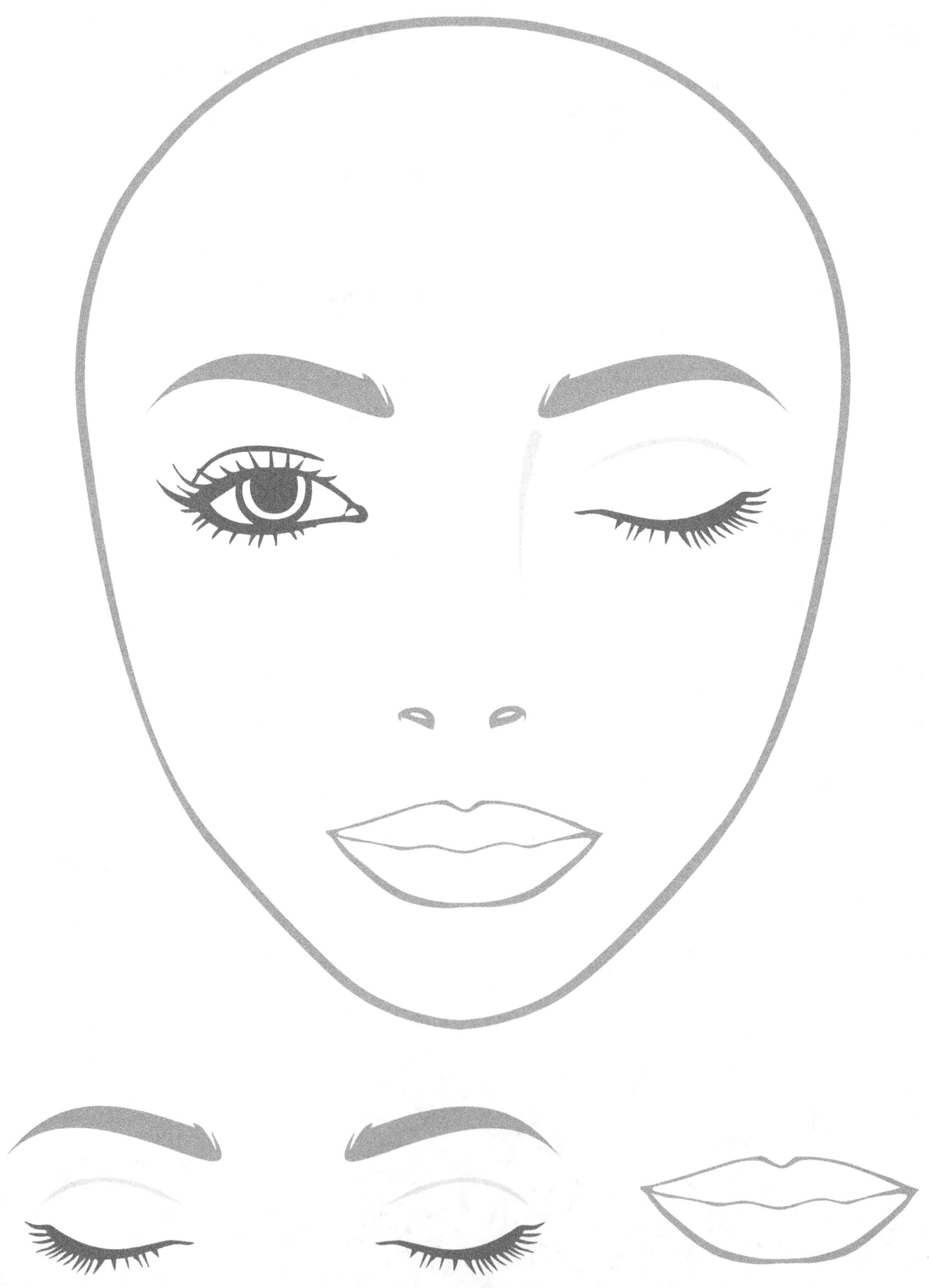

LOOK NAME _______________________   **FOR:** _______________________

◯ Daytime   ◯ Evening

FACE

Moisturizer

____

Primer

____

Powder

____

Highlight/Blush

____

Concealer

____

Foundation

____

Contour

____

EYES

Brows

____

Eyelid

____

Liner

____

Crease

____

Mascara

____

LIPS

Liner

____

Lip Color

____

Gloss

____

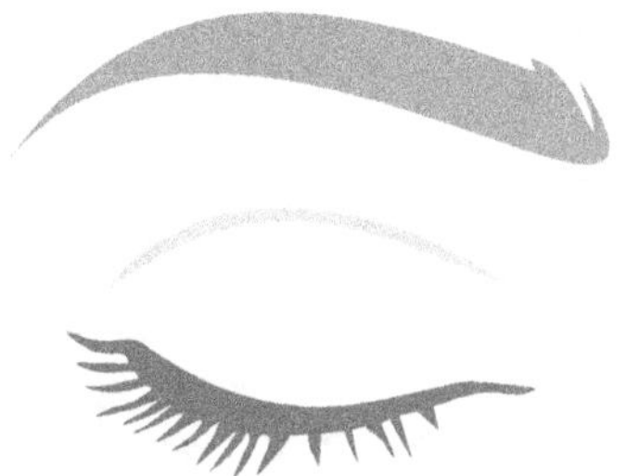
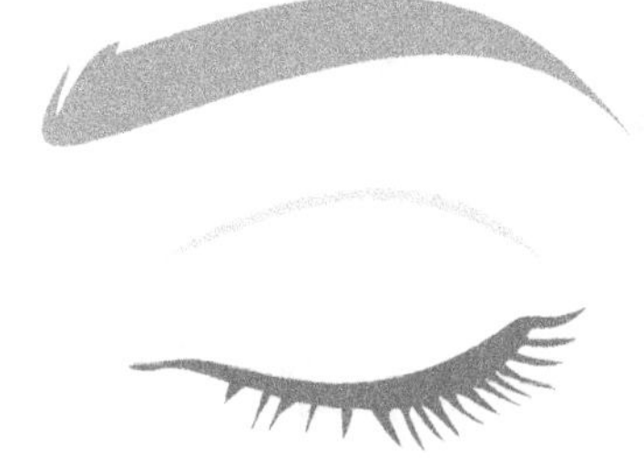
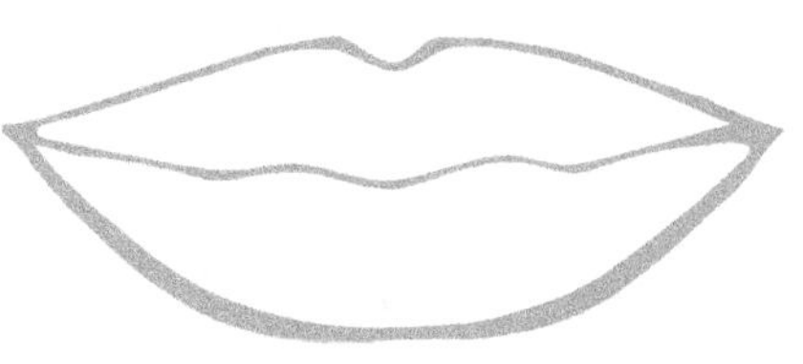

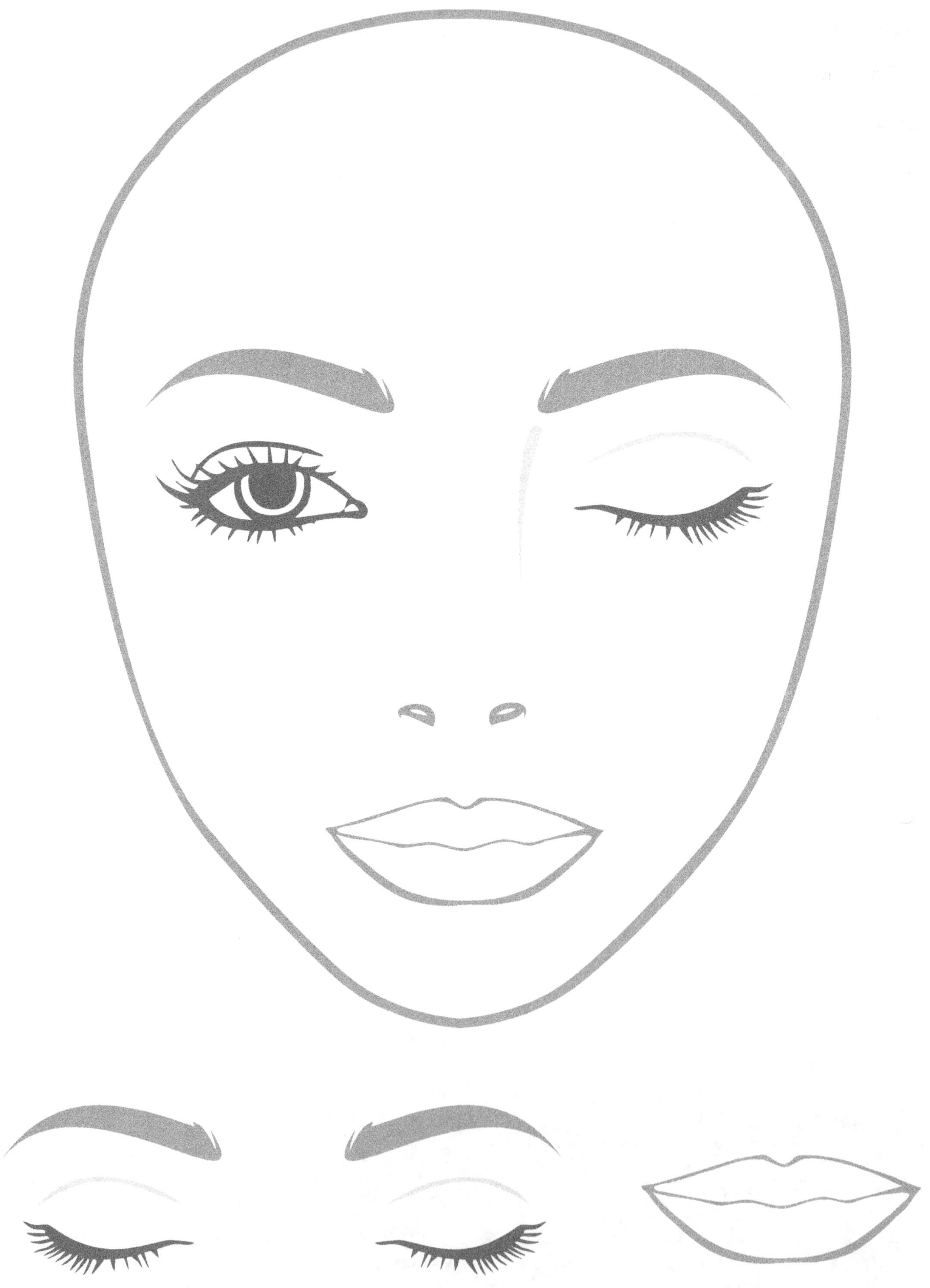

LOOK NAME _______________   FOR: _______________

○ Daytime   ○ Evening

FACE

Moisturizer

____

Primer

____

Powder

____

Highlight/Blush

____

Concealer

____

Foundation

____

Contour

____

EYES

Brows	Crease

Eyelid   Mascara

Liner

LIPS

Liner

Lip Color

Gloss

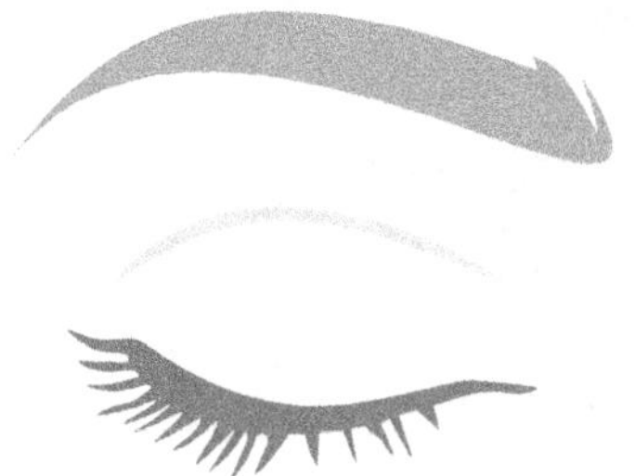

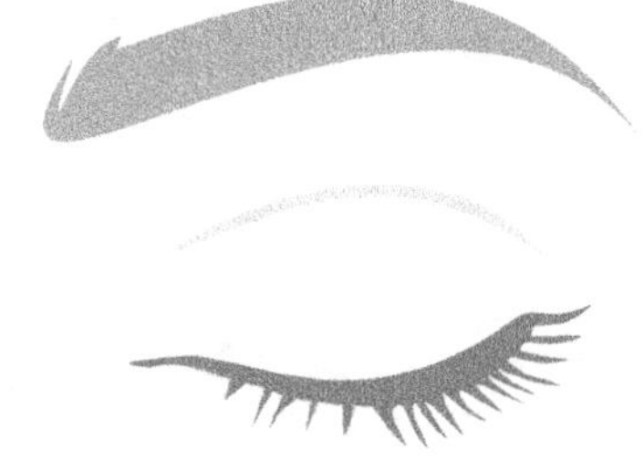

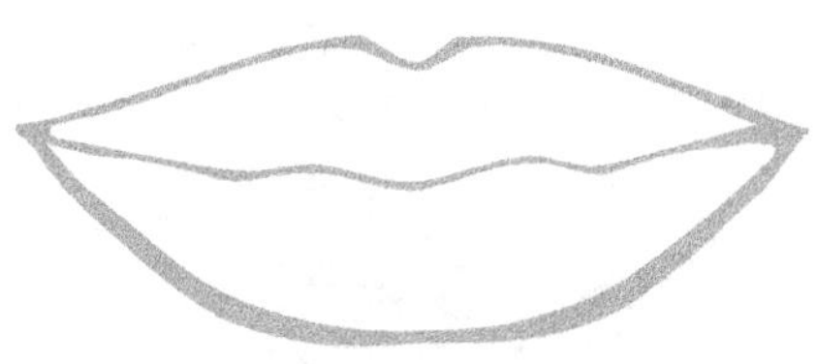

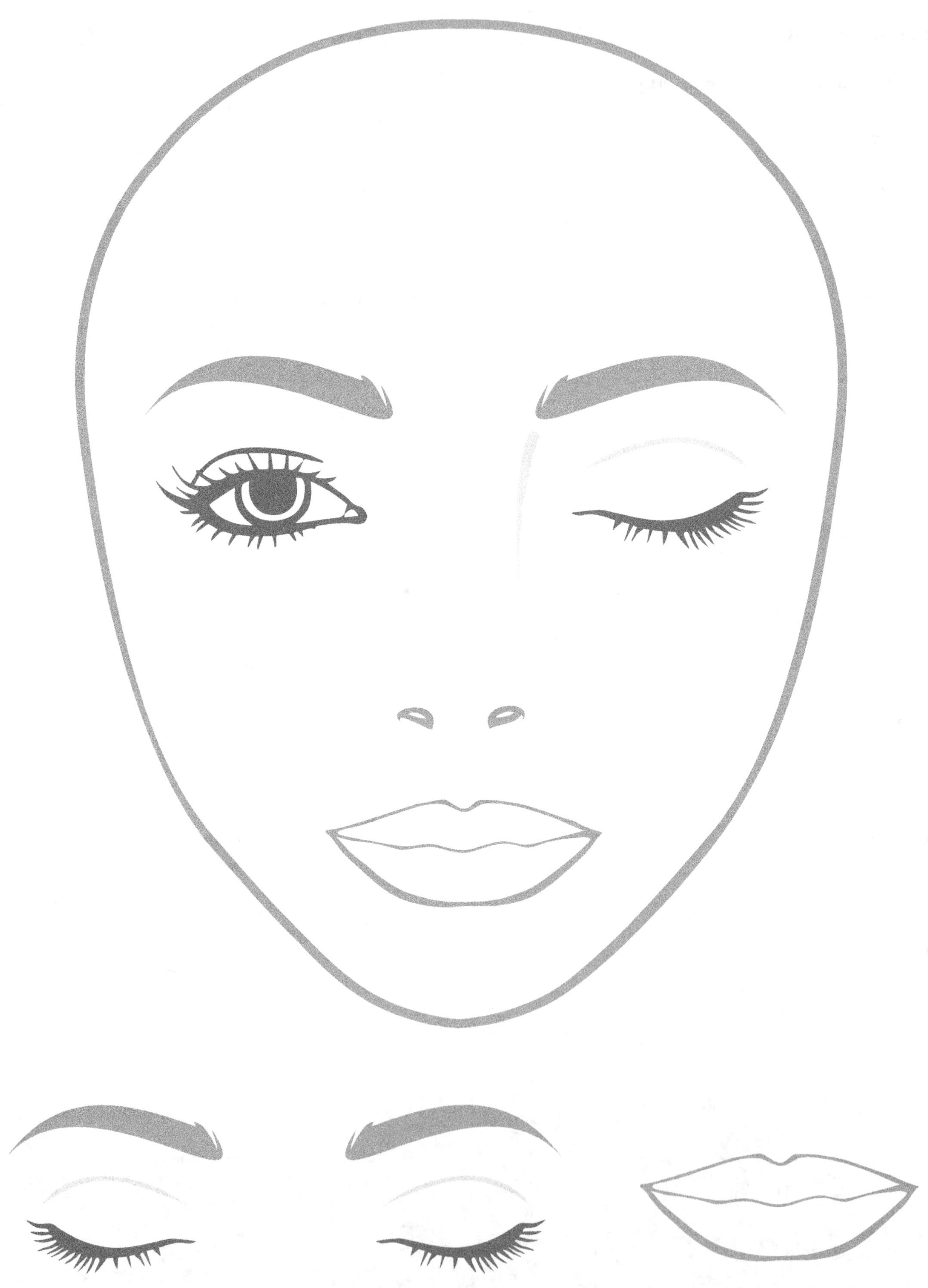

LOOK NAME _________________________   **FOR:** _________________________

◯ Daytime   ◯ Evening

FACE

Moisturizer

____

Primer

____

Powder

____

Highlight/Blush

____

Concealer

____

Foundation

____

Contour

____

EYES

Brows

____

Eyelid

____

Liner

____

Crease

____

Mascara

____

LIPS

Liner

____

Lip Color

____

Gloss

____

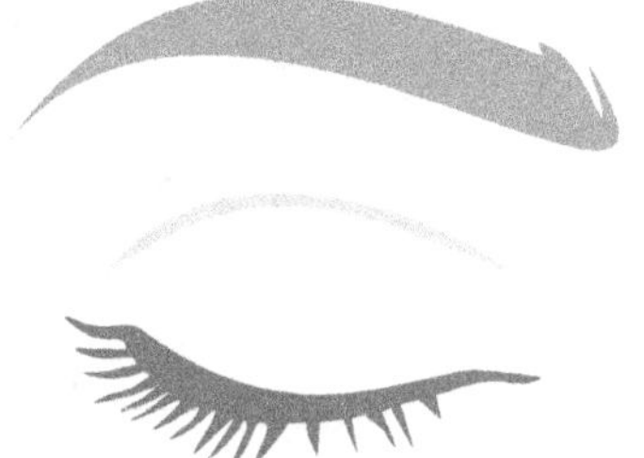
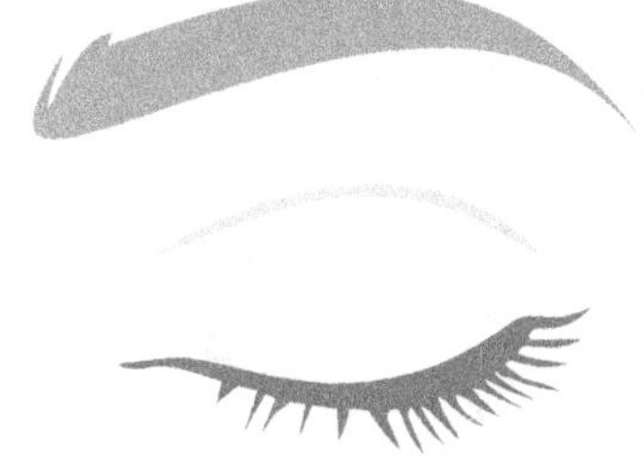
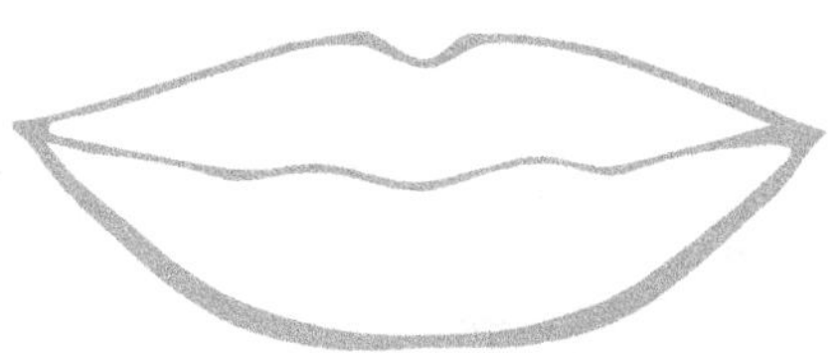

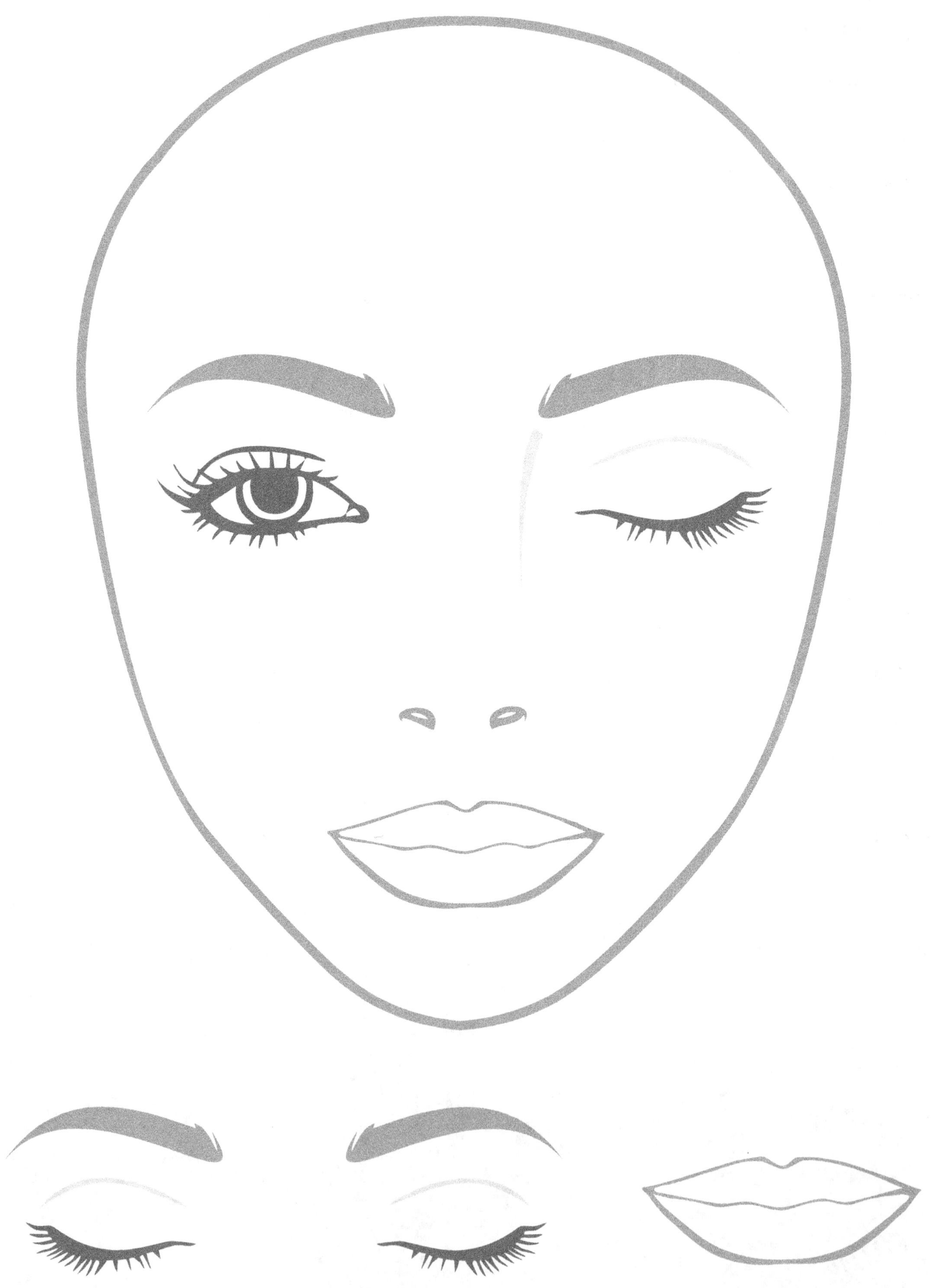

LOOK NAME ________________________   **FOR:** ________________________

◯ Daytime   ◯ Evening

FACE

Moisturizer

____

Primer

____

Powder

____

Highlight/Blush

____

Concealer

____

Foundation

____

Contour

____

EYES

Brows

____

Eyelid

____

Liner

____

Crease

____

Mascara

____

LIPS

Liner

____

Lip Color

____

Gloss

____

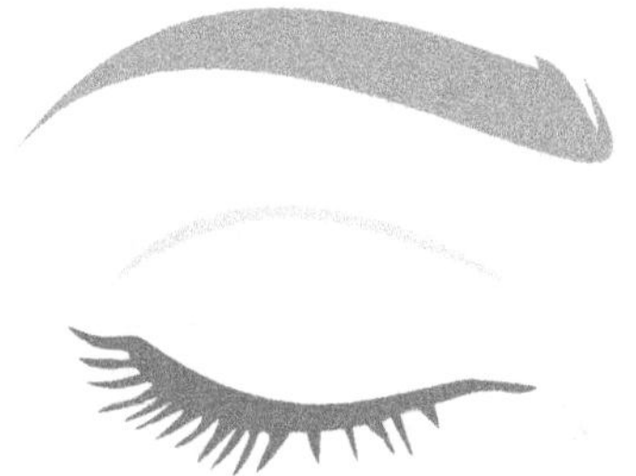
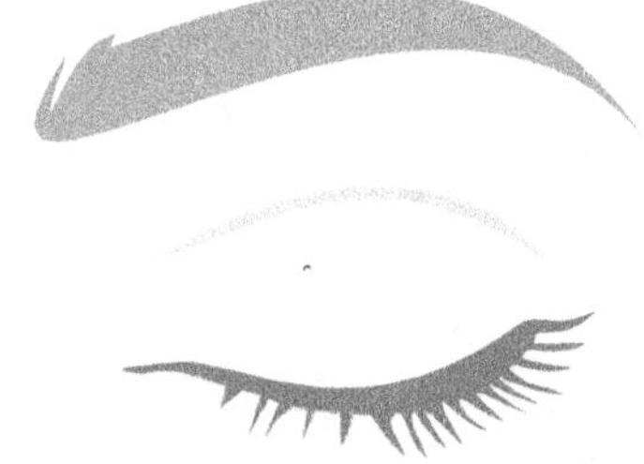
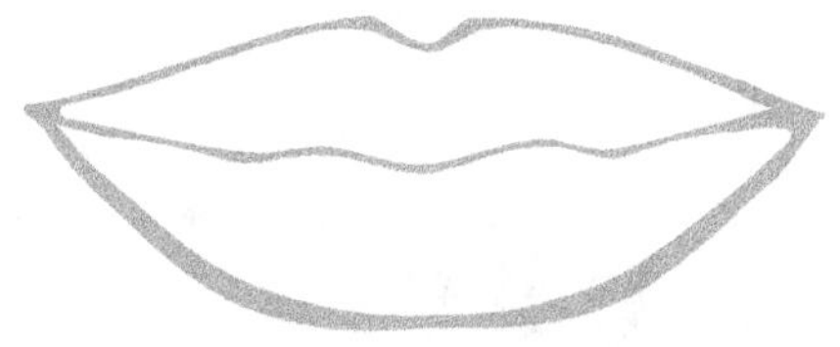

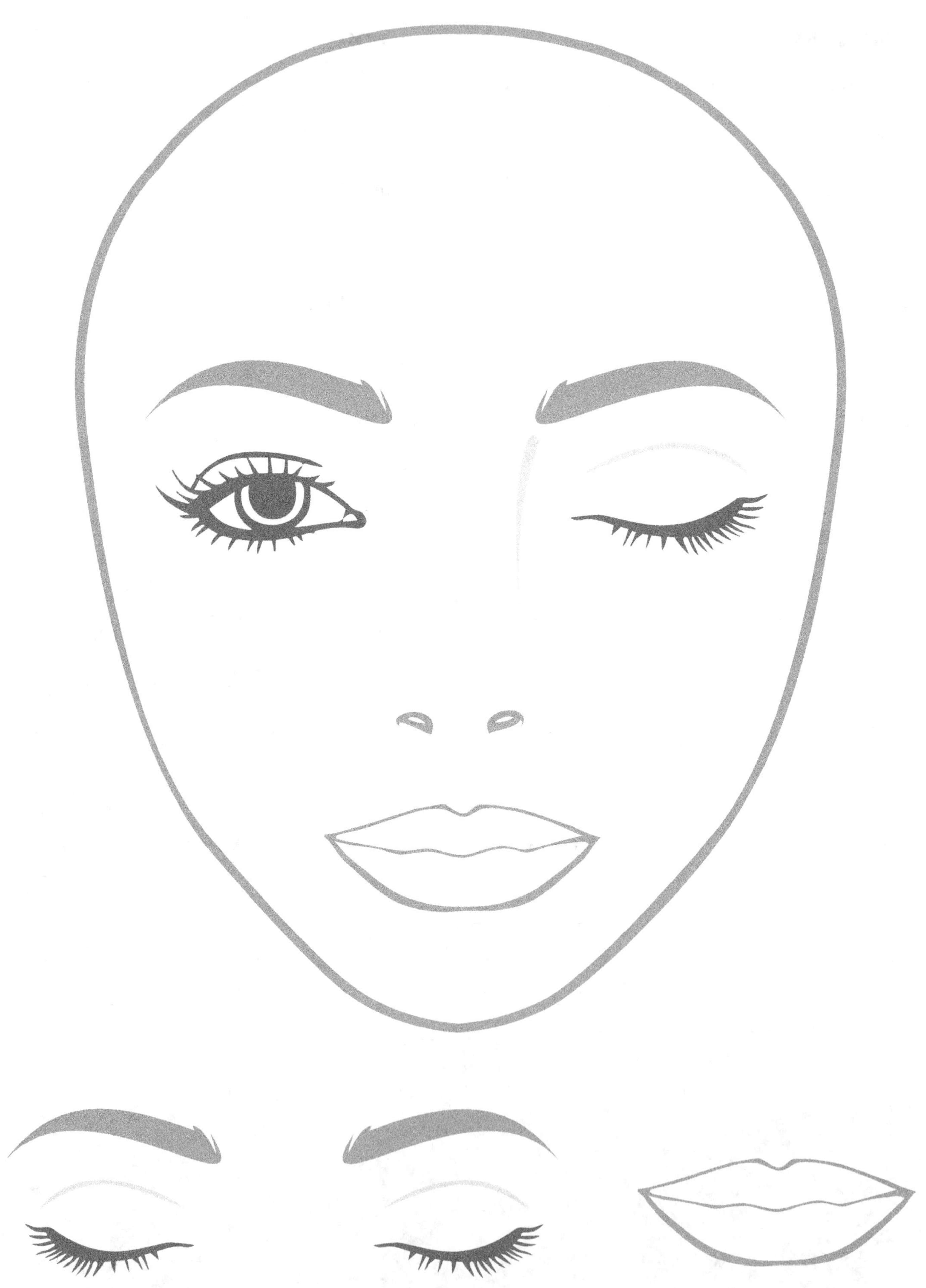

LOOK NAME _______________________   **FOR:** _______________________

◯ Daytime   ◯ Evening

FACE

Moisturizer

____

Primer

____

Powder

____

Highlight/Blush

____

Concealer

____

Foundation

____

Contour

____

EYES

Brows

____

Eyelid

____

Liner

____

Crease

____

Mascara

____

LIPS

Liner

____

Lip Color

____

Gloss

____

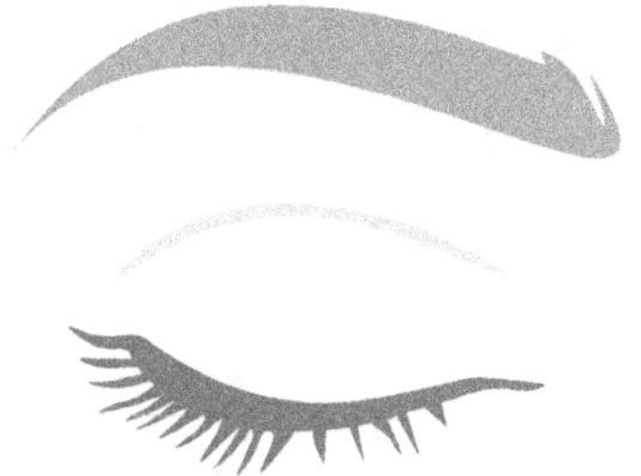
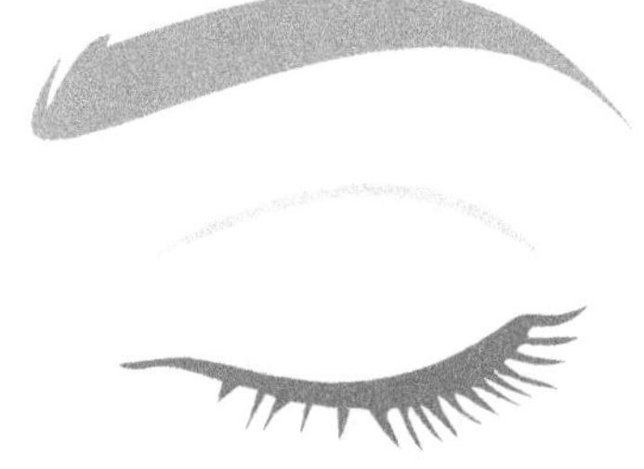
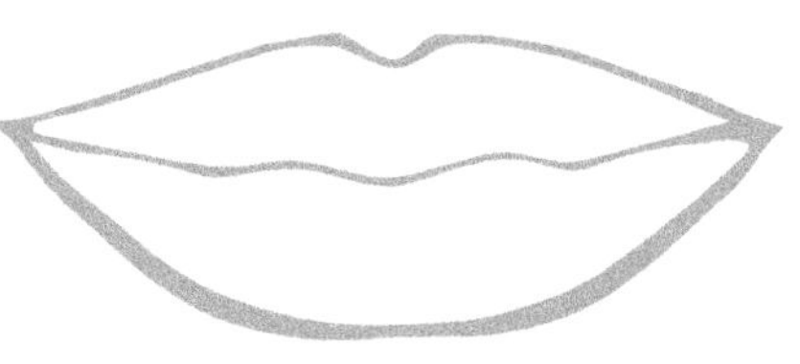

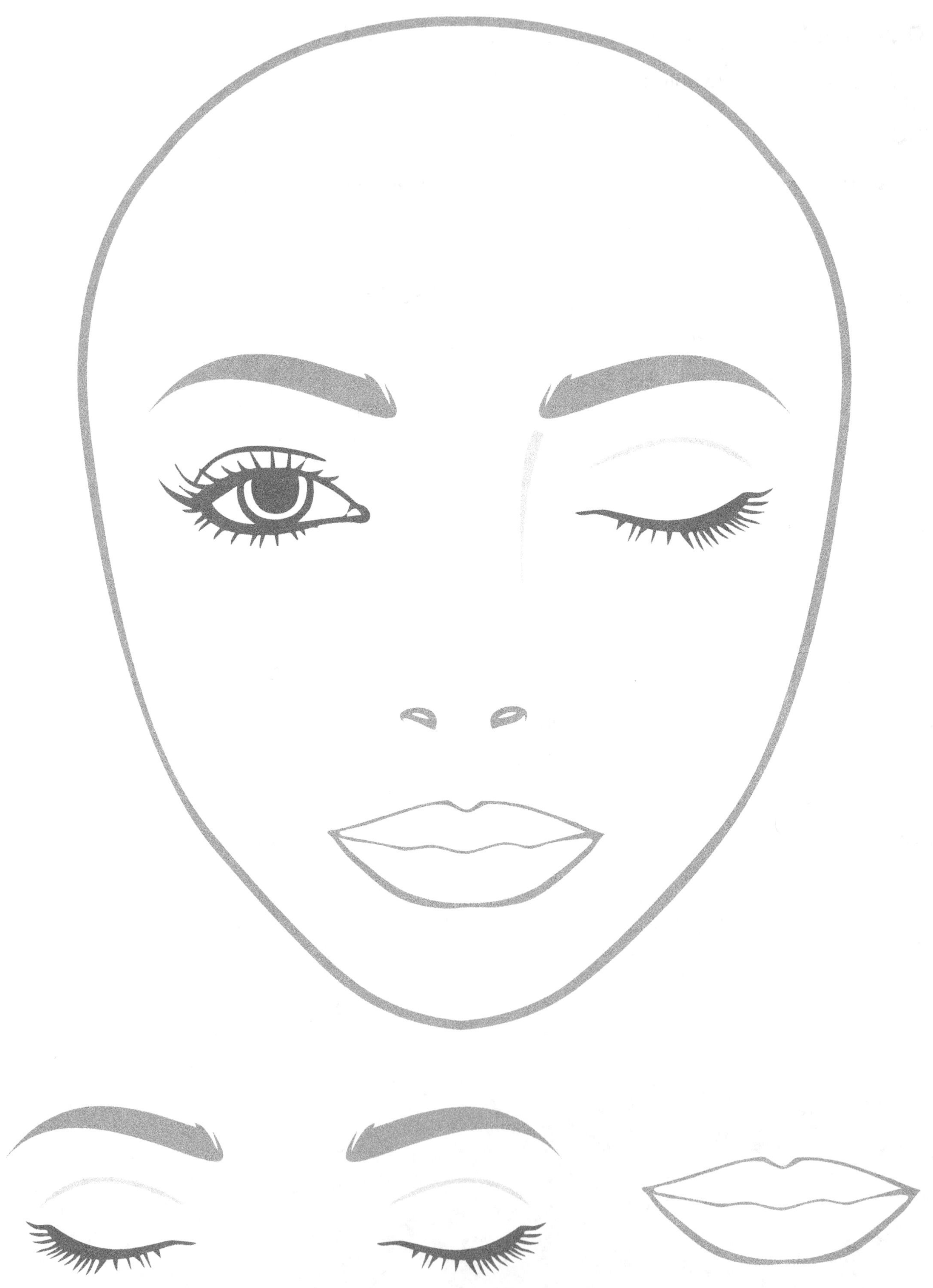

LOOK NAME ___________________________   FOR: ___________________

◯ Daytime   ◯ Evening

FACE

Moisturizer

____

Primer

____

Powder

____

Highlight/Blush

____

Concealer

____

Foundation

____

Contour

____

EYES

Brows

____

Eyelid

____

Liner

____

Crease

____

Mascara

____

LIPS

Liner

____

Lip Color

____

Gloss

____

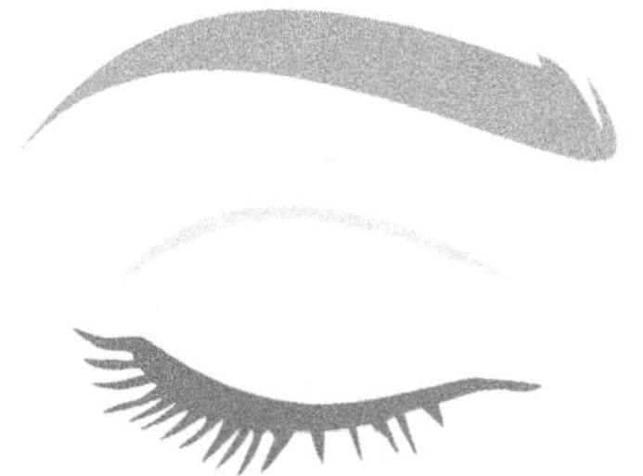

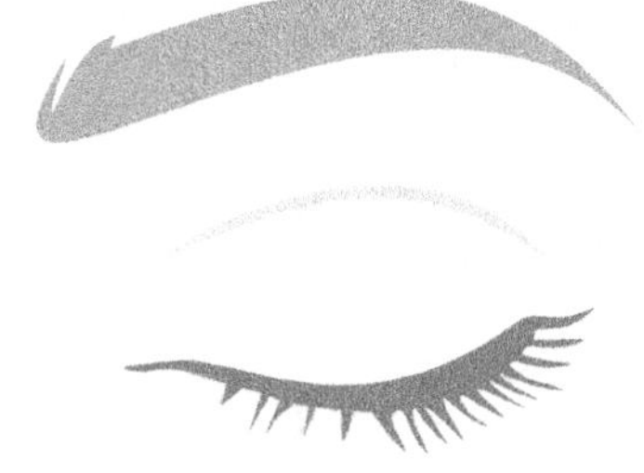

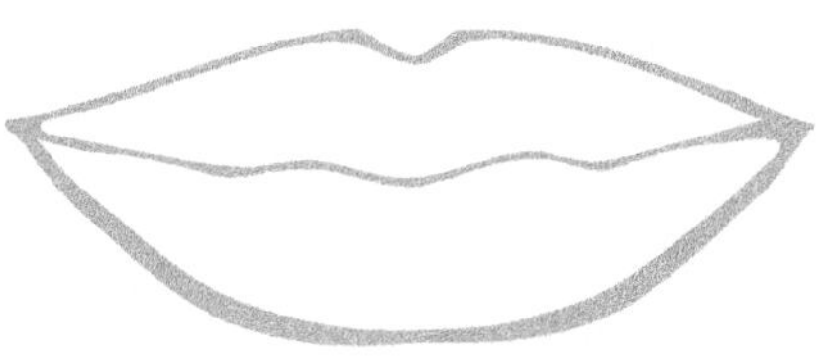

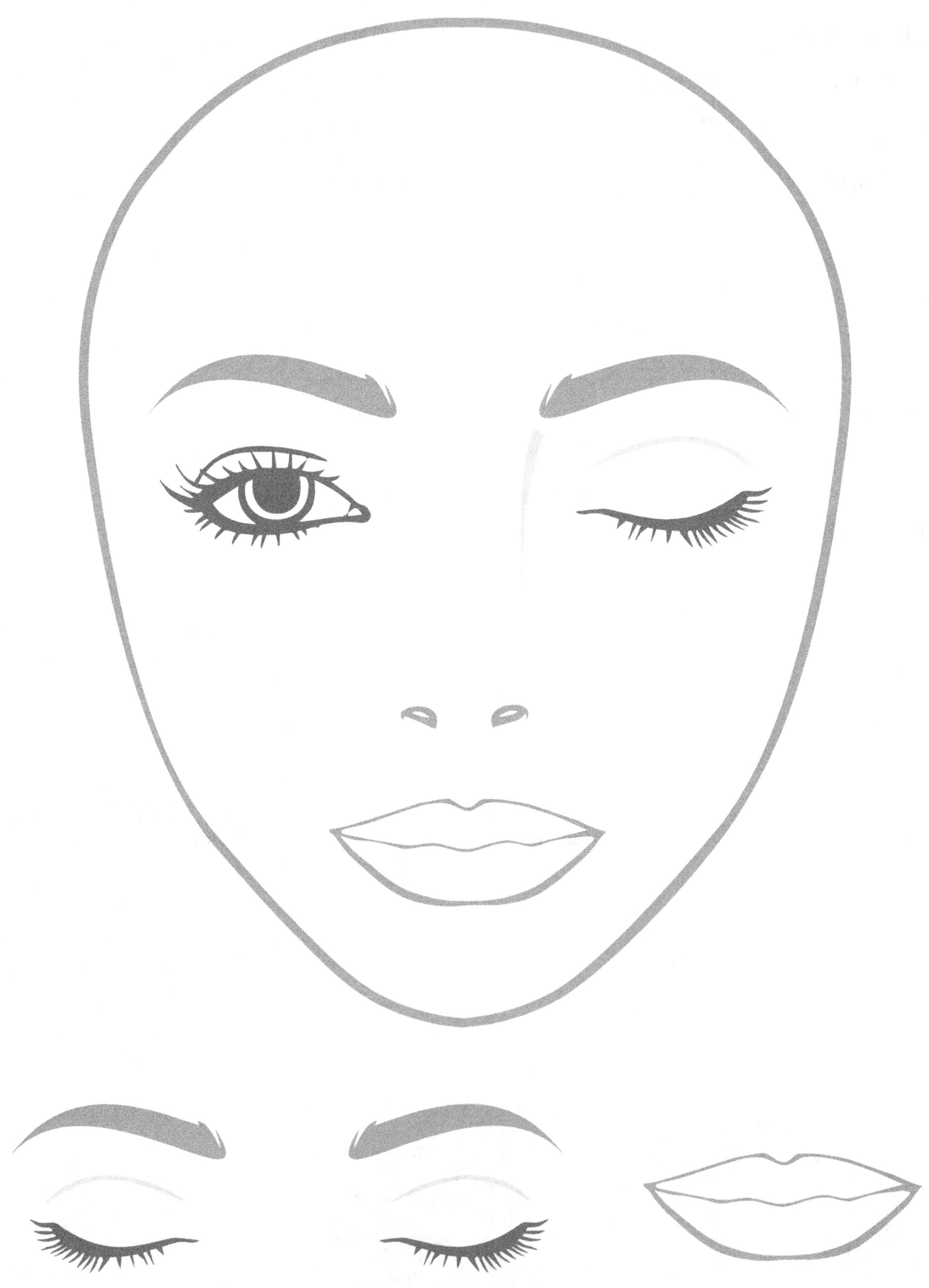

LOOK NAME ______________________   **FOR:** ______________________

◯ Daytime   ◯ Evening

FACE

Moisturizer

____

Primer

____

Powder

____

Highlight/Blush

____

Concealer

____

Foundation

____

Contour

____

EYES

Brows   Crease

____

Eyelid   Mascara

____

Liner

____

LIPS

Liner

____

Lip Color

____

Gloss

____

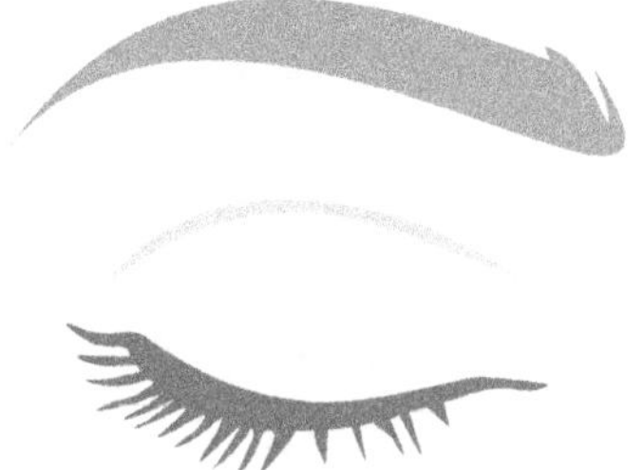
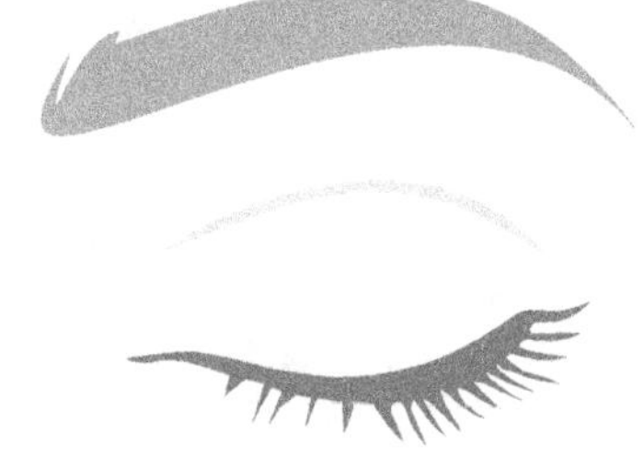
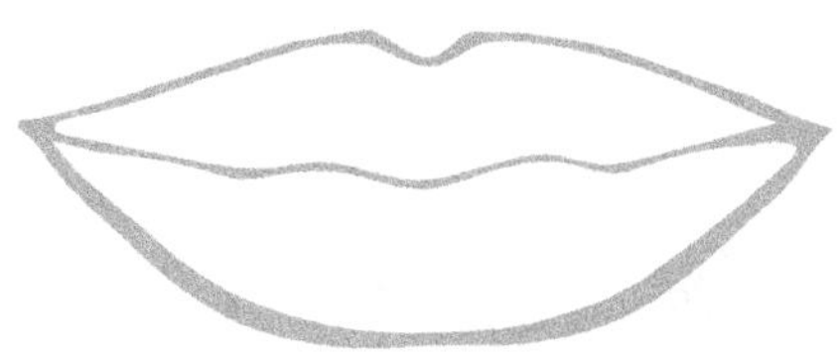

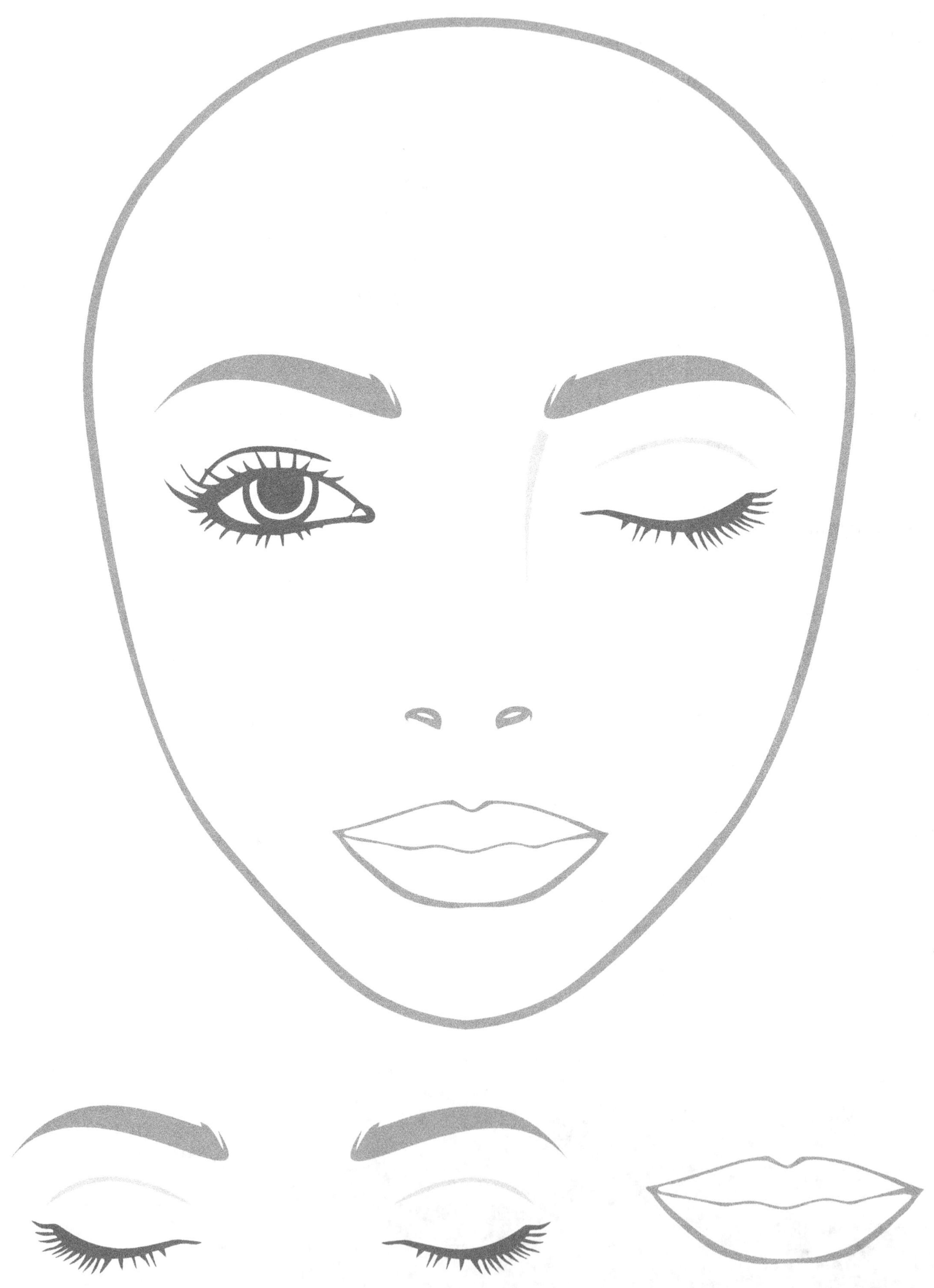

LOOK NAME ______________________________   **FOR:** ______________________________

◯ Daytime   ◯ Evening

FACE

Moisturizer

____

Primer

____

Powder

____

Highlight/Blush

____

Concealer

____

Foundation

____

Contour

____

EYES

Brows

____

Eyelid

____

Liner

____

Crease

____

Mascara

____

LIPS

Liner

____

Lip Color

____

Gloss

____

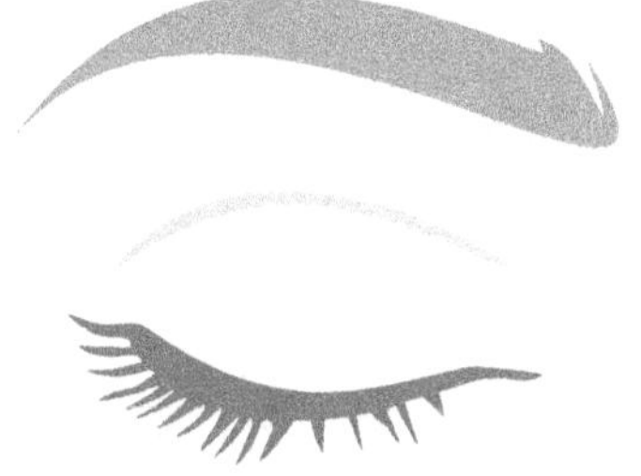
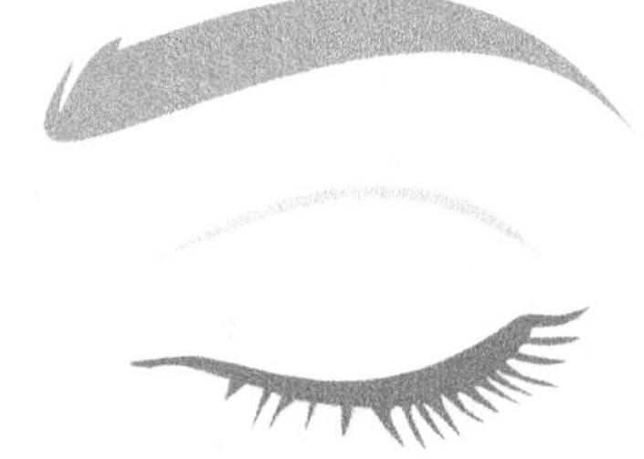
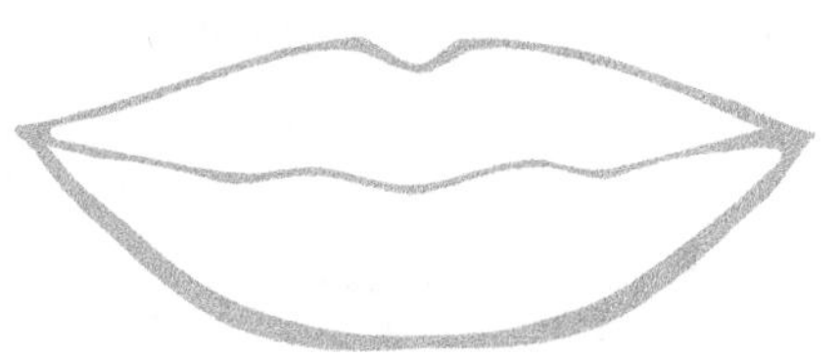

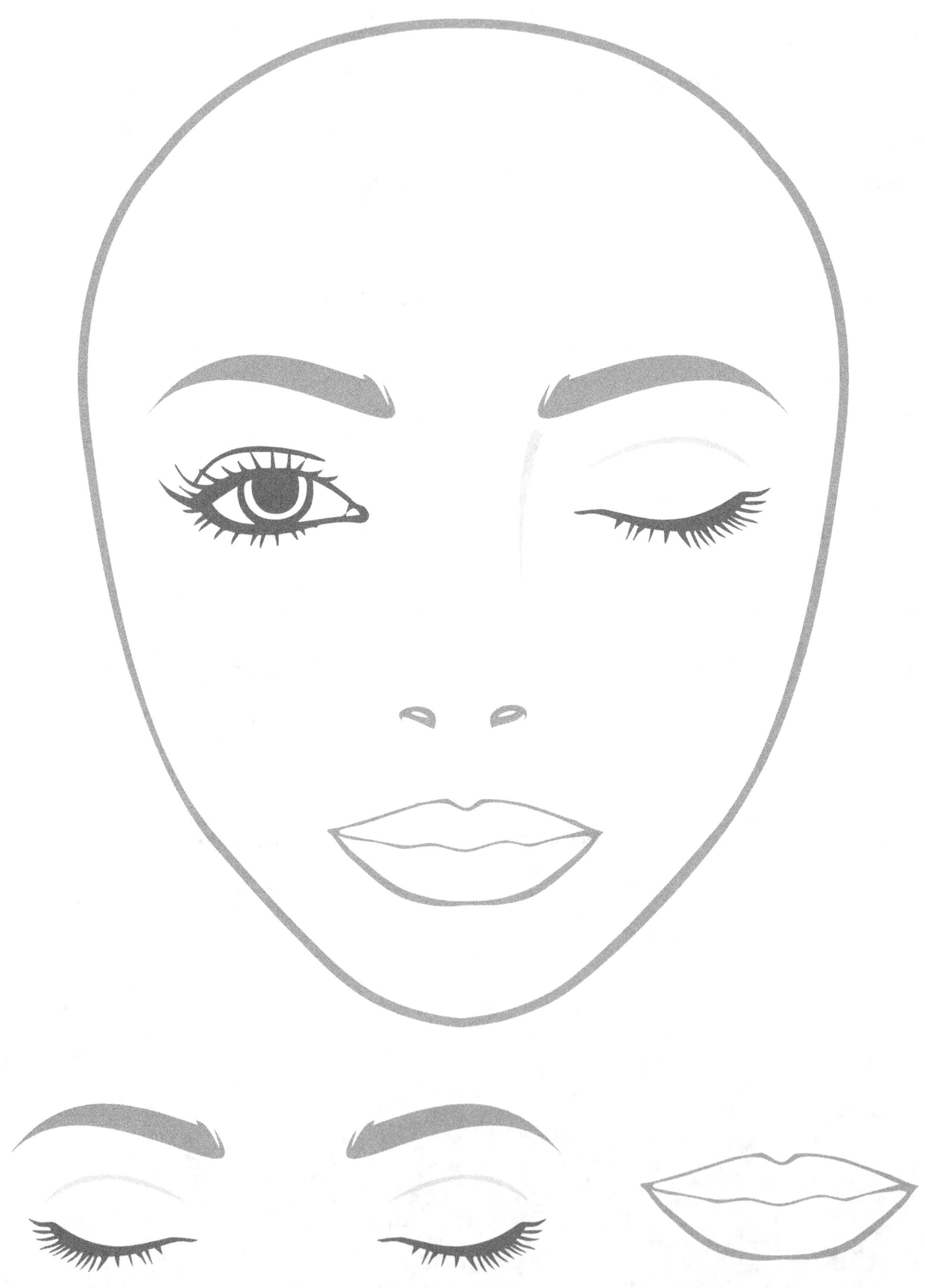

LOOK NAME _______________________   FOR: _______________________

◯ Daytime   ◯ Evening

FACE

Moisturizer

____

Primer

____

Powder

____

Highlight/Blush

____

Concealer

____

Foundation

____

Contour

____

EYES

Brows

____

Eyelid

____

Liner

____

Crease

____

Mascara

LIPS

Liner

____

Lip Color

____

Gloss

____

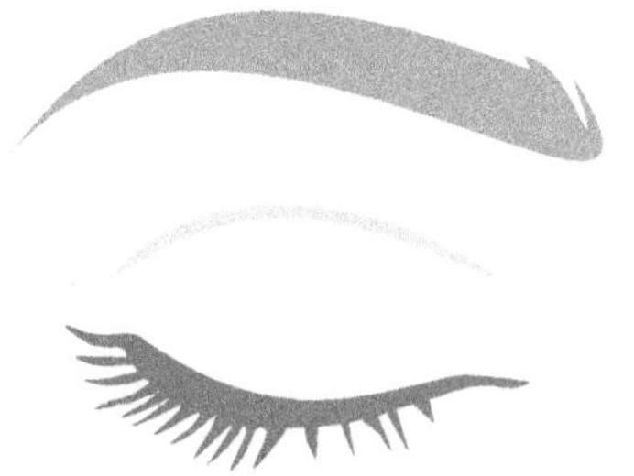

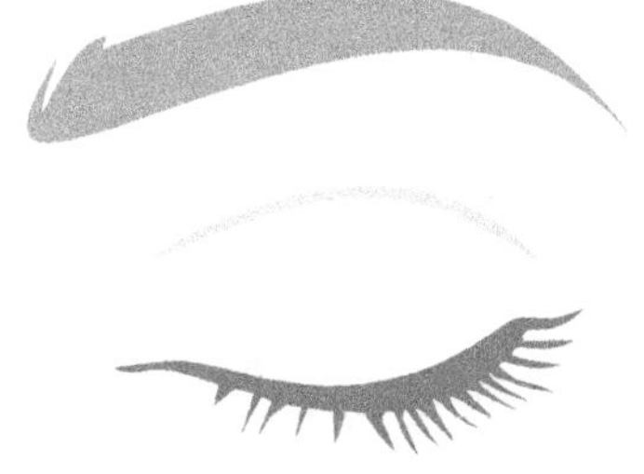

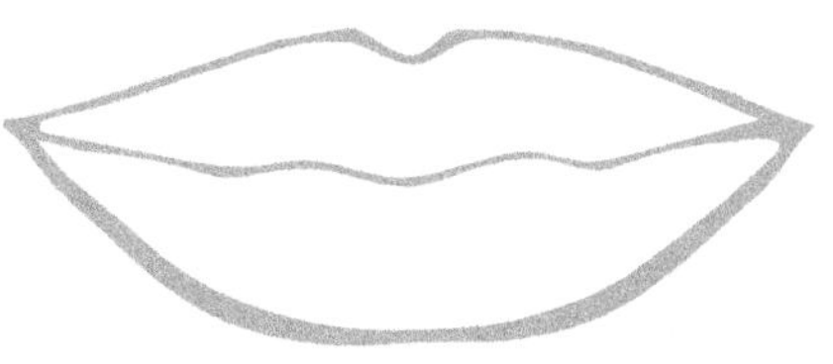

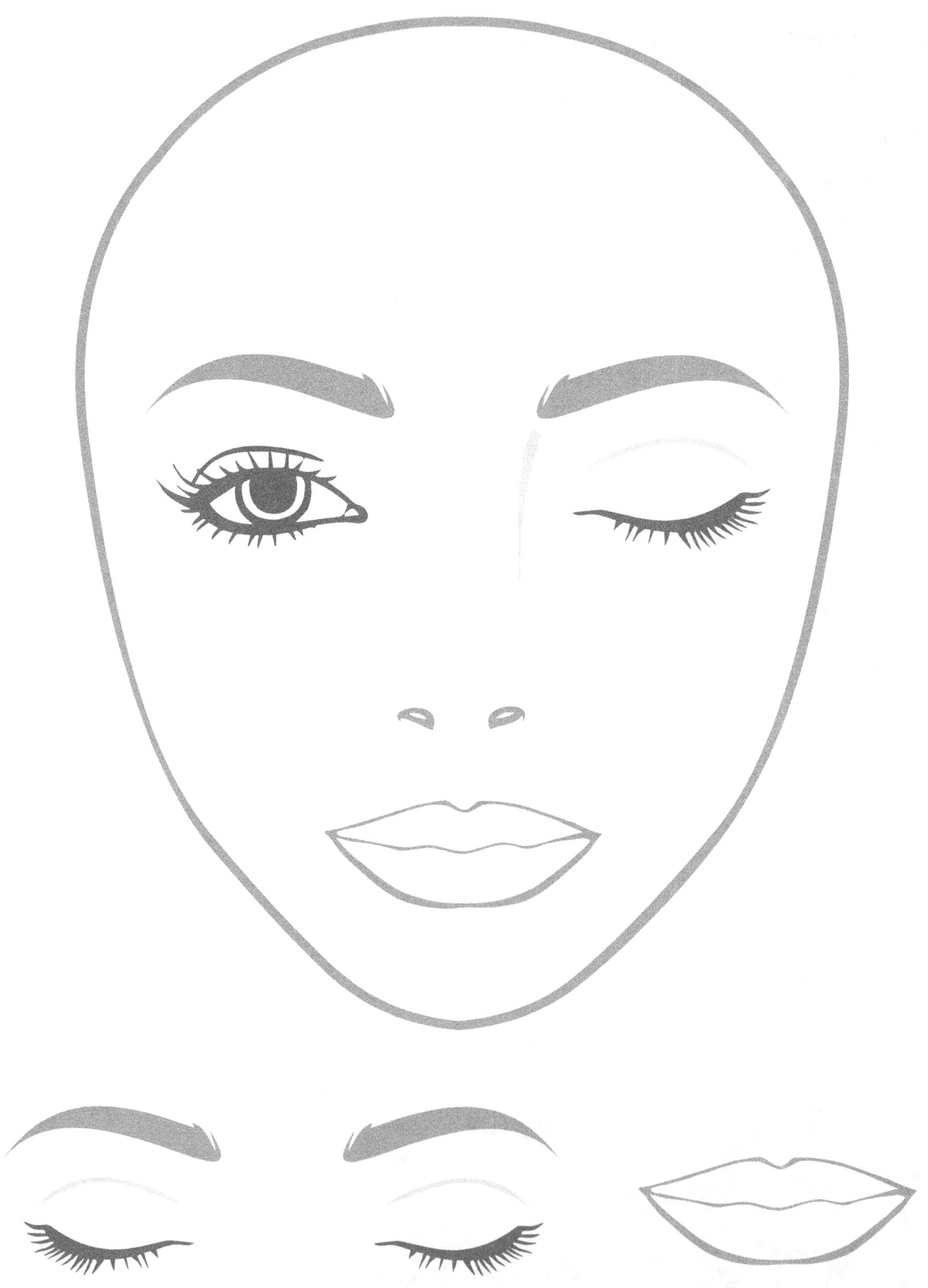

LOOK NAME __________________   FOR: __________________

◯ Daytime   ◯ Evening

FACE

Moisturizer

____

Primer

____

Powder

____

Highlight/Blush

____

Concealer

____

Foundation

____

Contour

____

EYES

Brows

____

Eyelid

____

Liner

____

Crease

____

Mascara

____

LIPS

Liner

____

Lip Color

____

Gloss

____

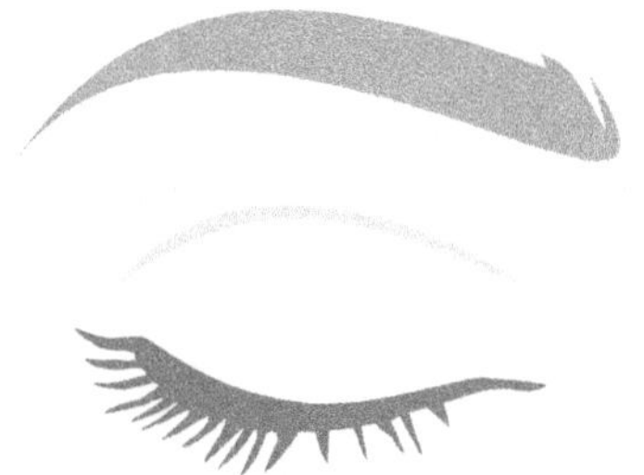
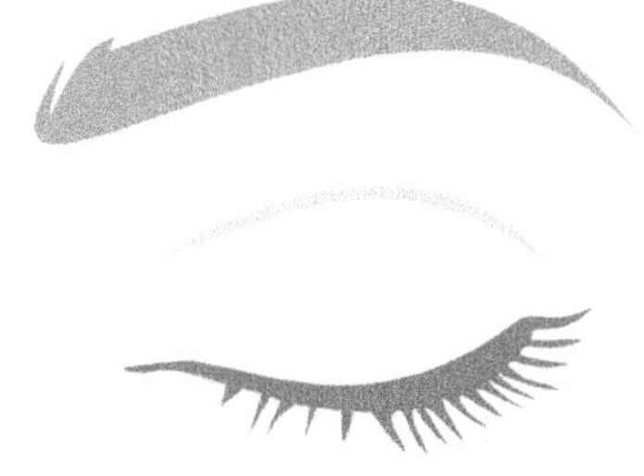
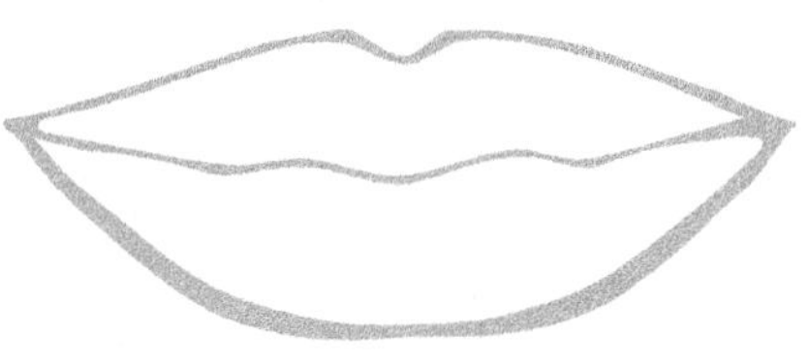

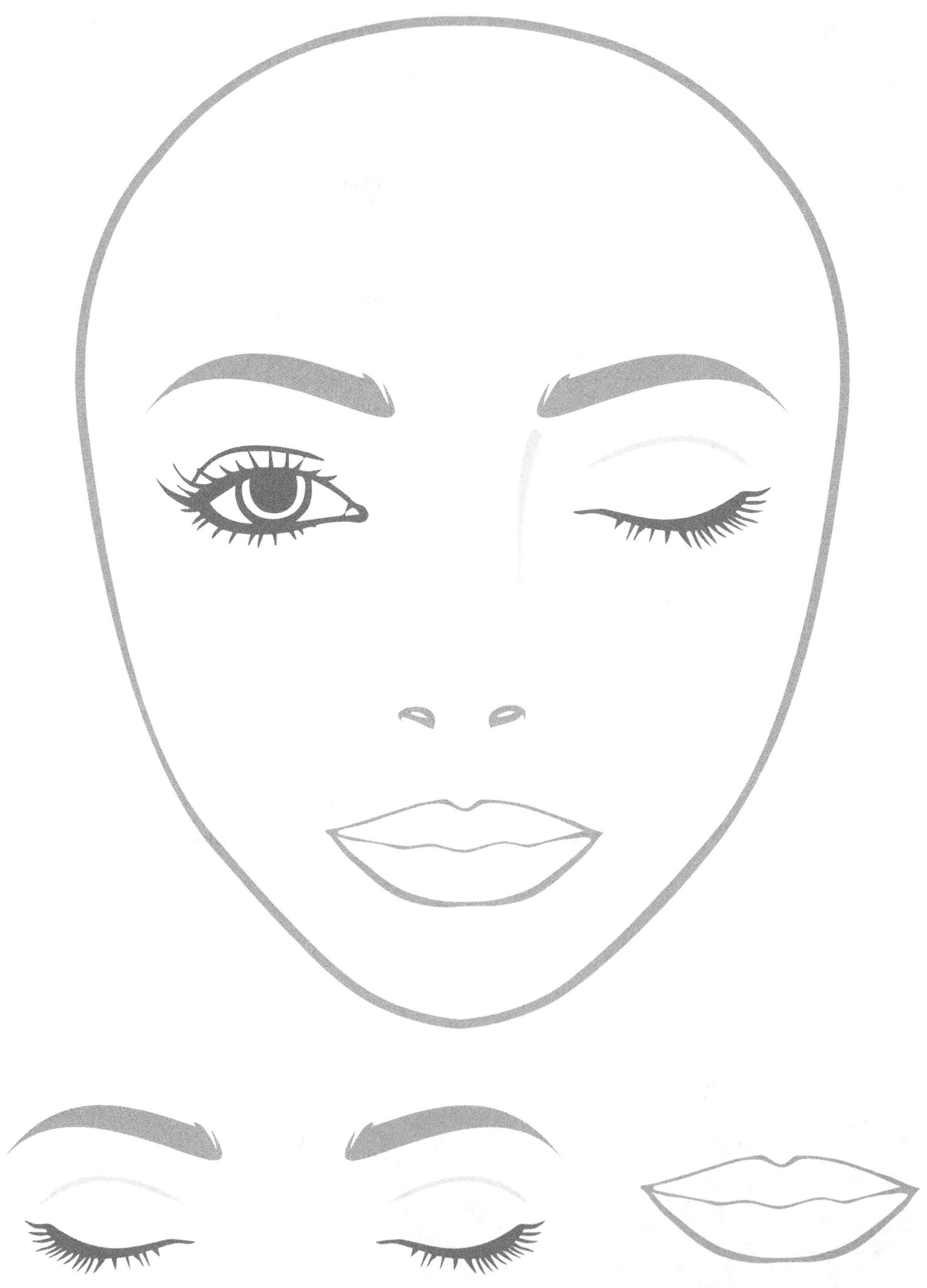

LOOK NAME ________________ FOR: ________________

◯ Daytime　　◯ Evening

FACE

Moisturizer

Primer

Powder

Highlight/Blush

Concealer

Foundation

Contour

EYES

Brows

Eyelid

Liner

Crease

Mascara

LIPS

Liner

Lip Color

Gloss

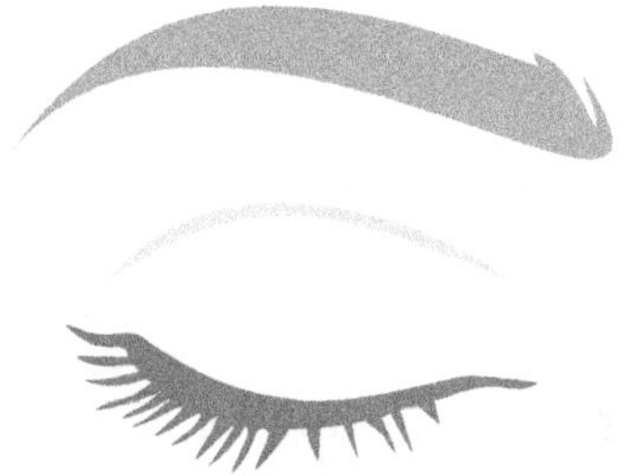

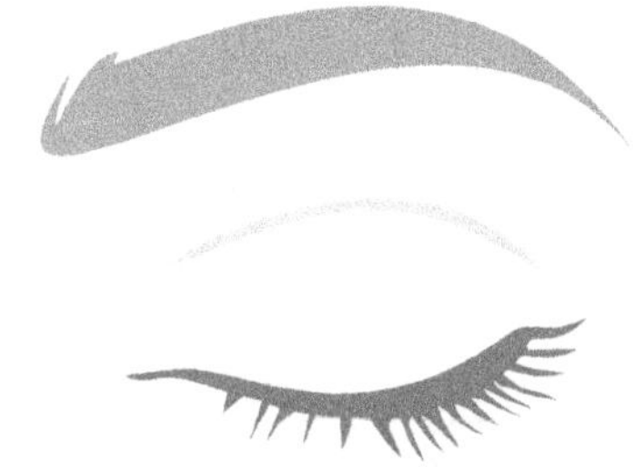

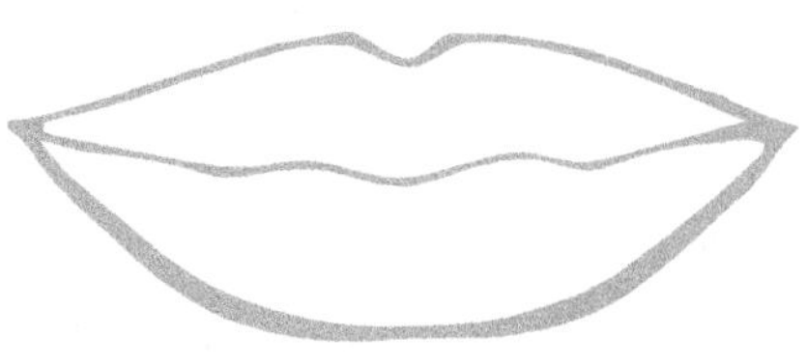

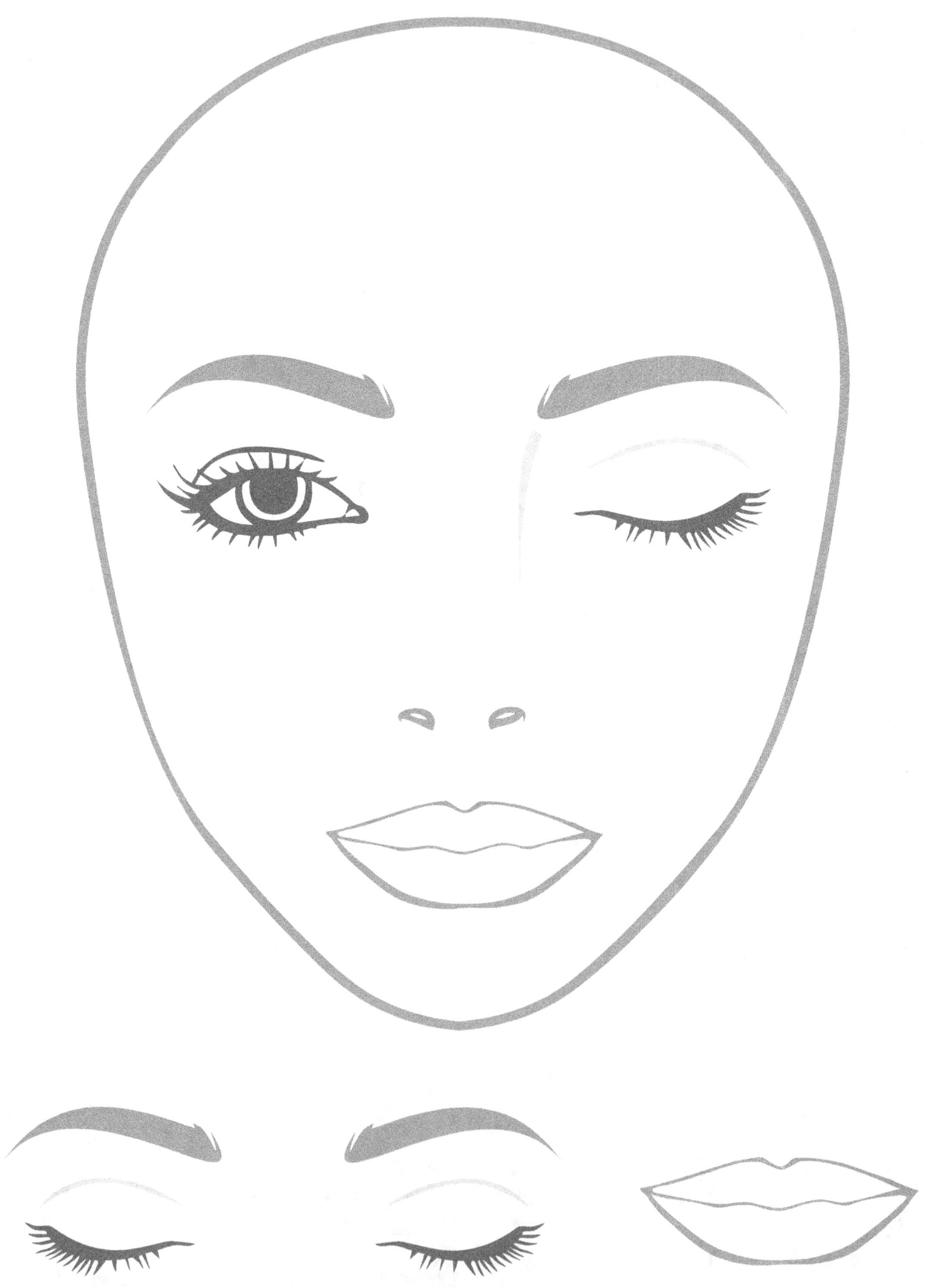

LOOK NAME ______________________   FOR: ______________________

◯ Daytime   ◯ Evening

FACE

Moisturizer

Primer

Powder

Highlight/Blush

Concealer

Foundation

Contour

EYES

Brows   Crease

Eyelid   Mascara

Liner

LIPS

Liner

Lip Color

Gloss

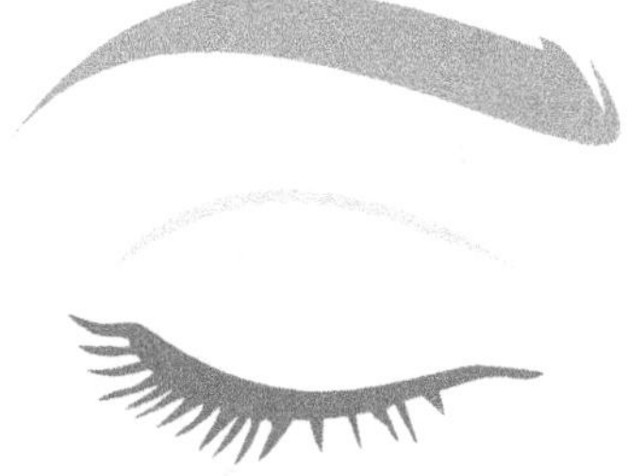

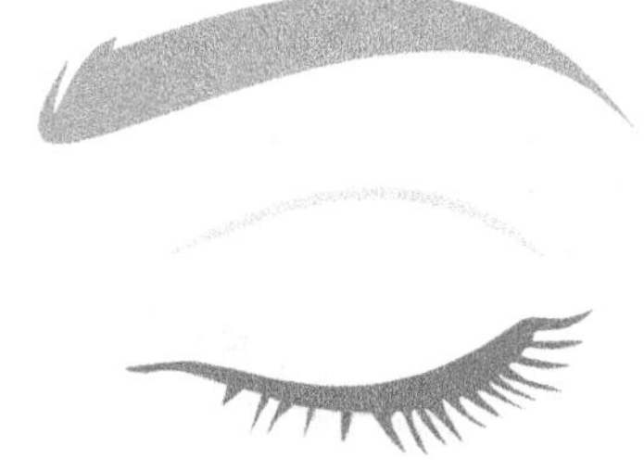

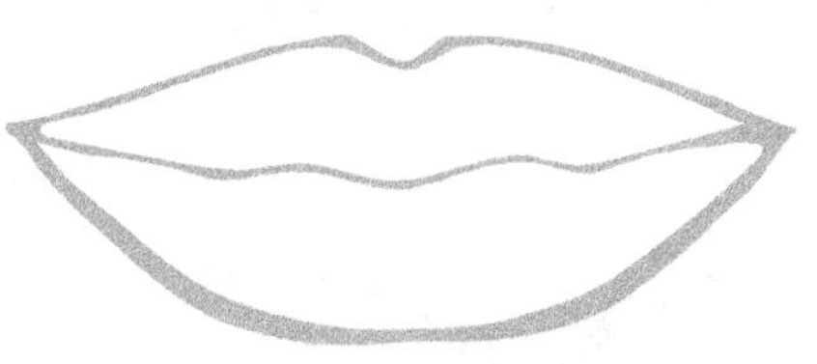

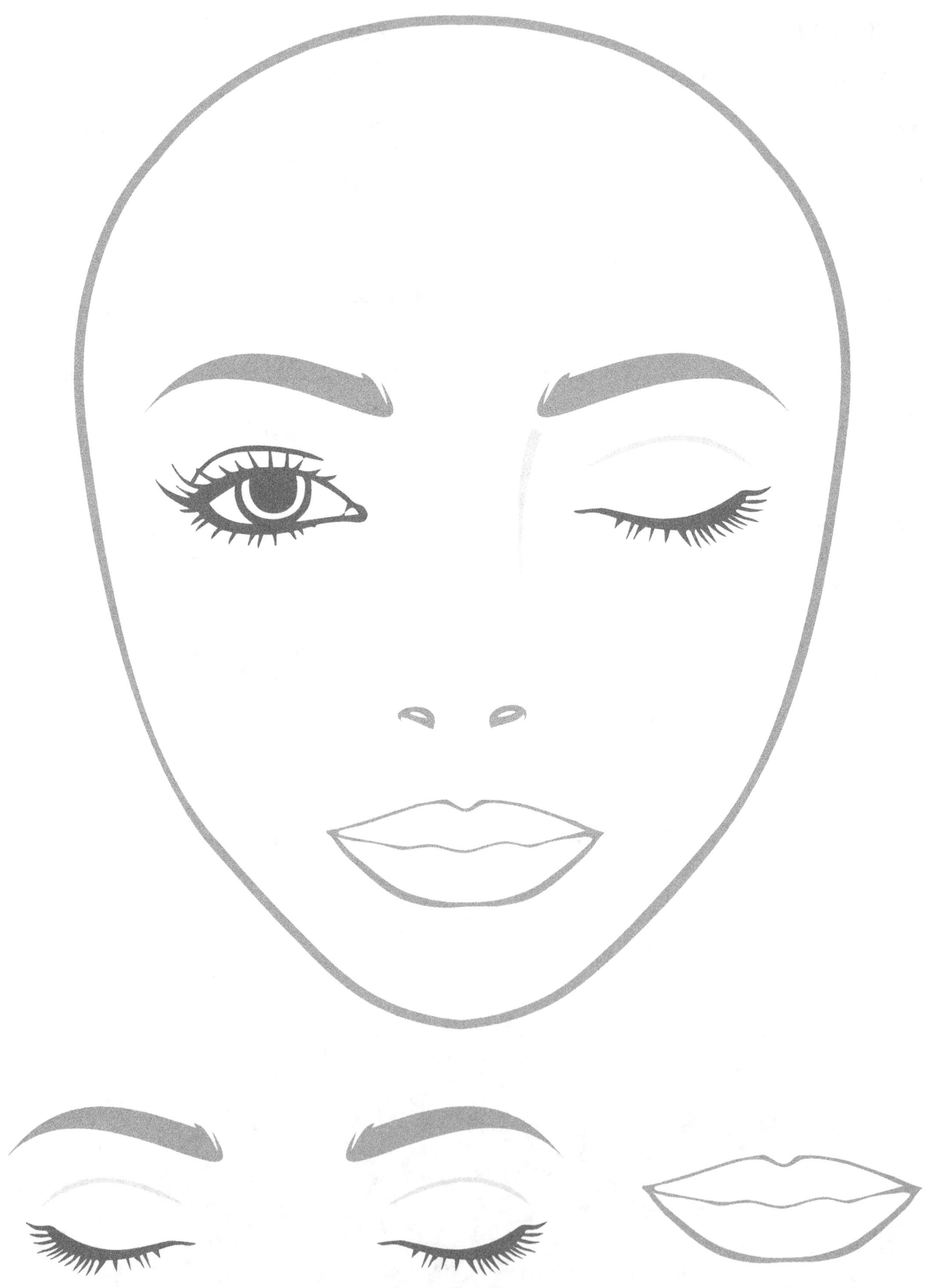

LOOK NAME _______________________________   **FOR:** _______________________________

◯ Daytime   ◯ Evening

FACE

Moisturizer

____

Primer

____

Powder

____

Highlight/Blush

____

Concealer

____

Foundation

____

Contour

____

EYES

Brows

____

Eyelid

____

Liner

____

Crease

____

Mascara

____

LIPS

Liner

____

Lip Color

____

Gloss

____

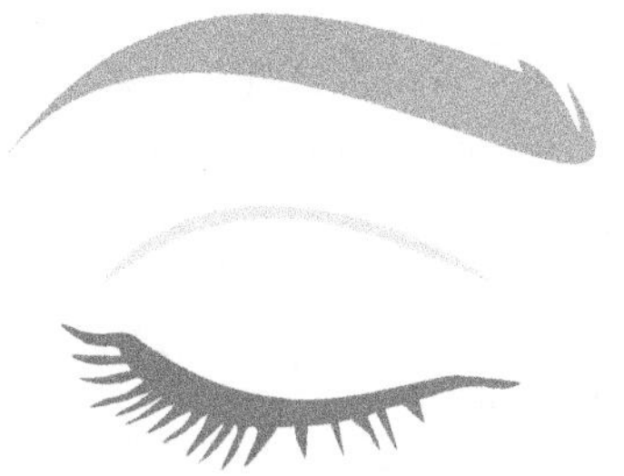
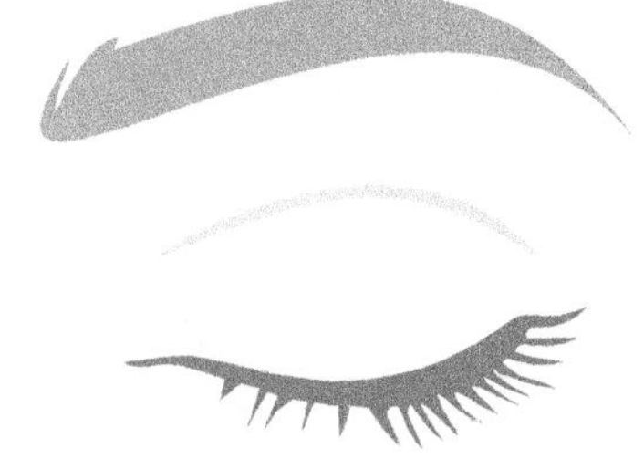
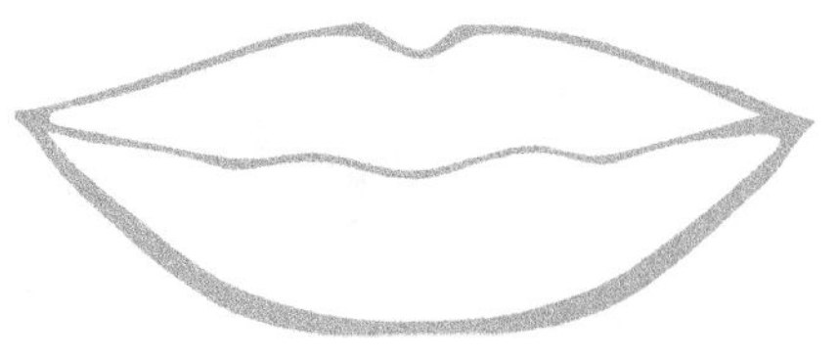

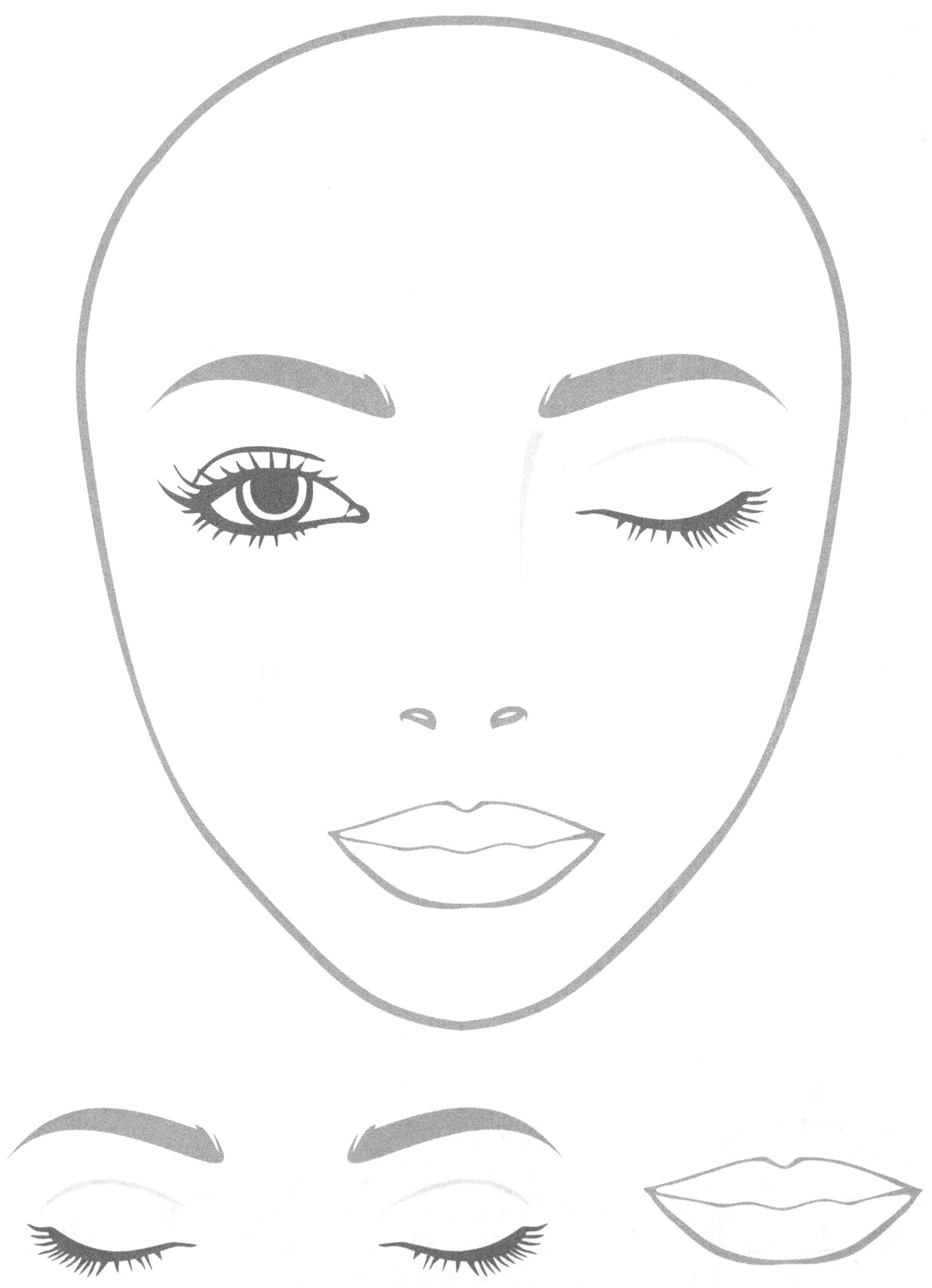

LOOK NAME ________________   FOR: ________________

◯ Daytime   ◯ Evening

FACE

Moisturizer

____

Primer

____

Powder

____

Highlight/Blush

____

Concealer

____

Foundation

____

Contour

____

EYES

Brows

____

Eyelid

____

Liner

____

Crease

____

Mascara

____

LIPS

Liner

____

Lip Color

____

Gloss

____

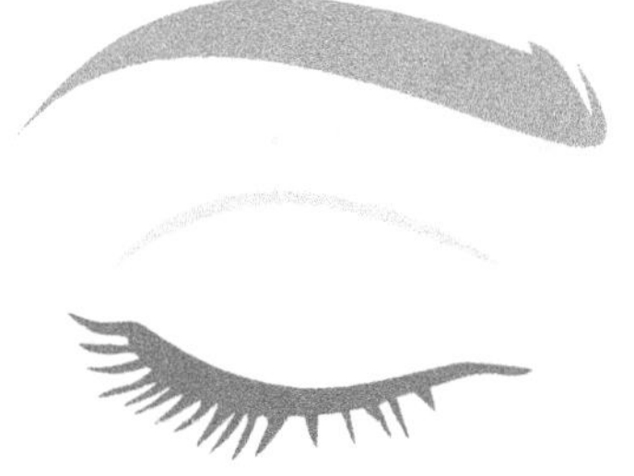
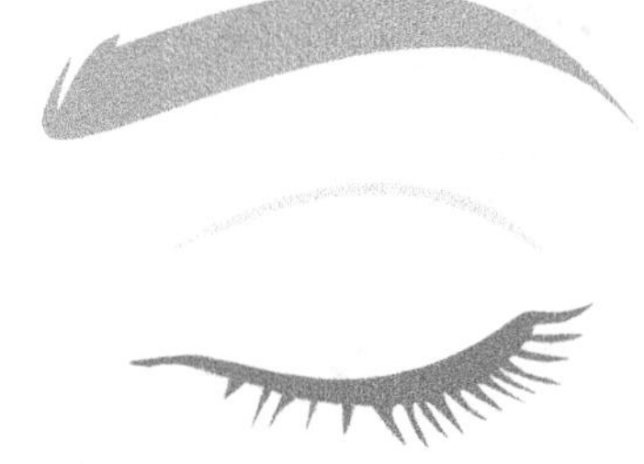
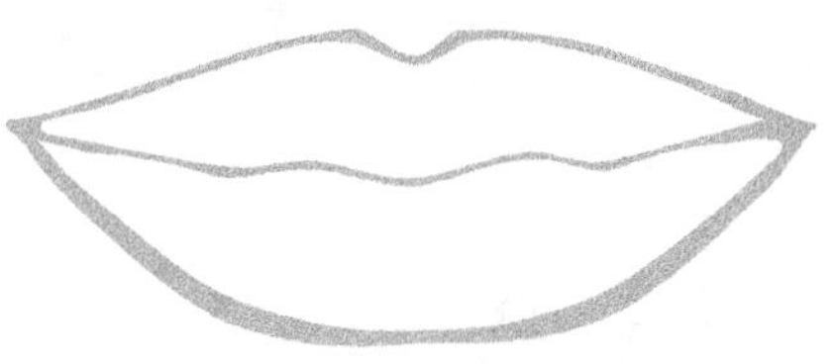

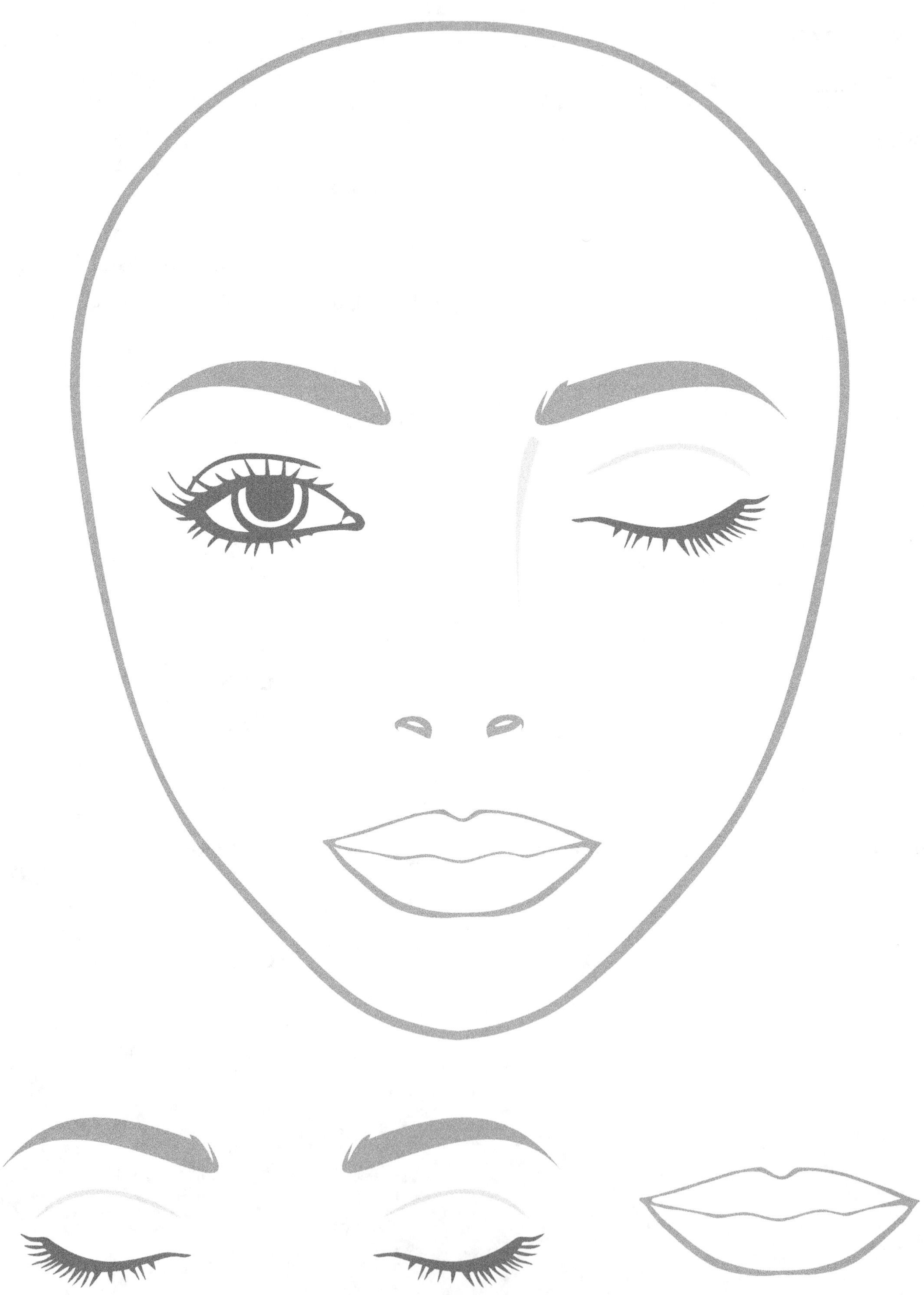

LOOK NAME _______________________   **FOR:** _______________________

◯ Daytime   ◯ Evening

FACE

Moisturizer

____

Primer

____

Powder

____

Highlight/Blush

____

Concealer

____

Foundation

____

Contour

____

EYES

Brows

____

Eyelid

____

Liner

____

Crease

____

Mascara

____

LIPS

Liner

____

Lip Color

____

Gloss

____

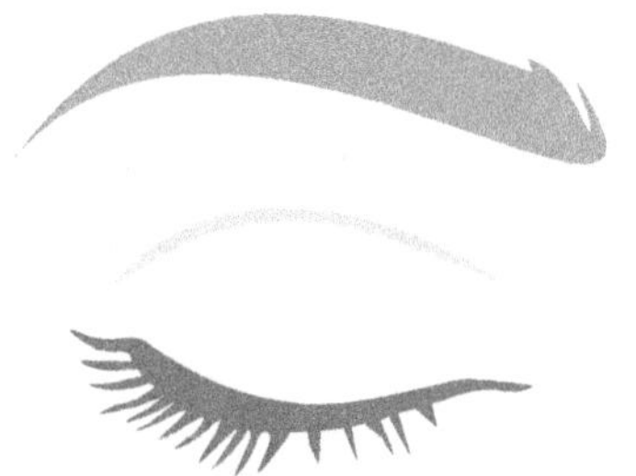
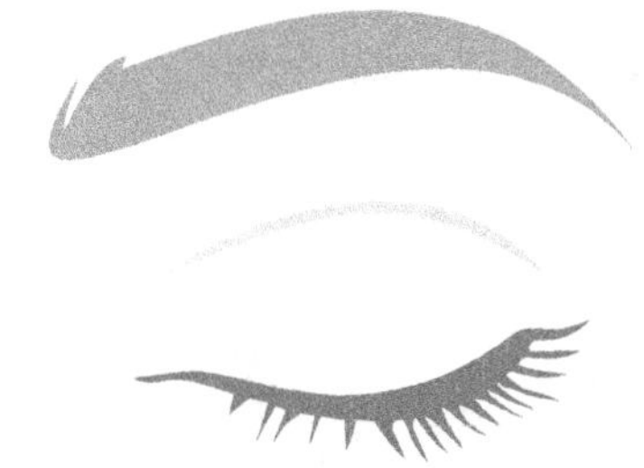
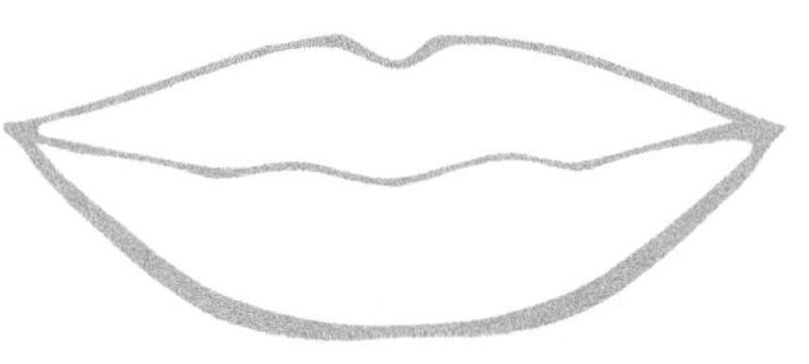

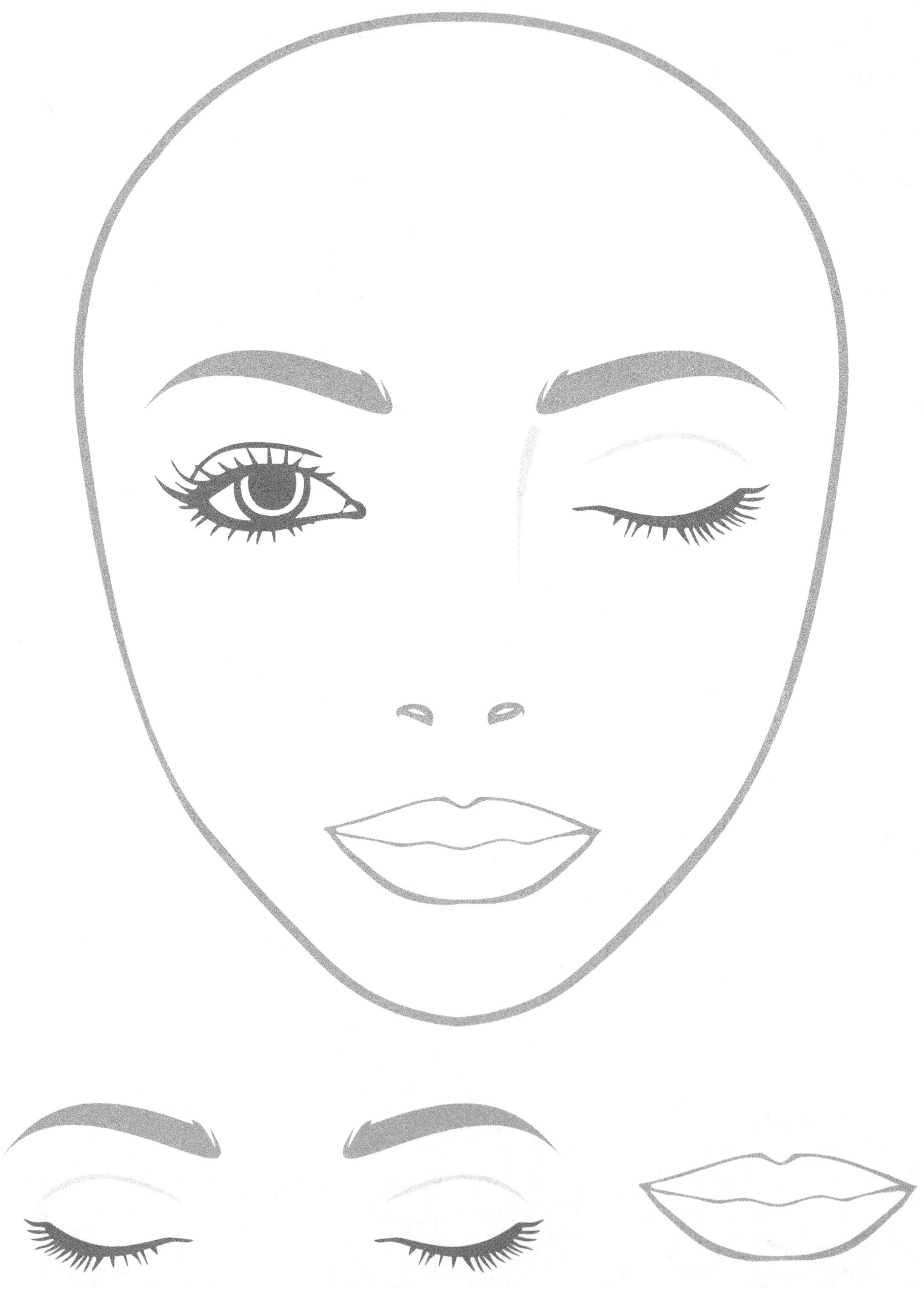

LOOK NAME _______________________ **FOR:** _______________________

◯ Daytime   ◯ Evening

FACE

Moisturizer

____

Primer

____

Powder

____

Highlight/Blush

____

Concealer

____

Foundation

____

Contour

____

EYES

Brows

____

Eyelid

____

Liner

____

Crease

____

Mascara

____

LIPS

Liner

____

Lip Color

____

Gloss

____

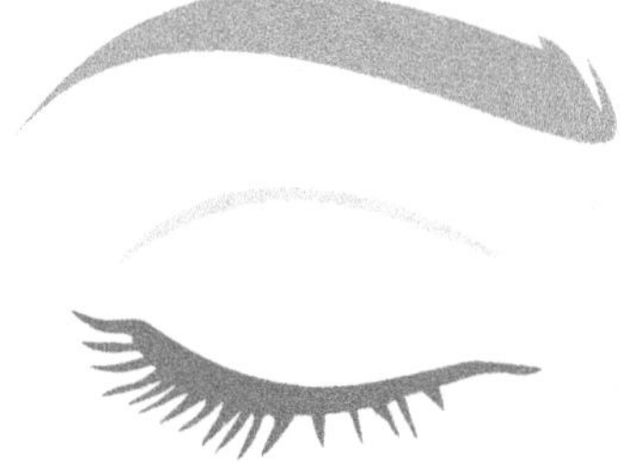
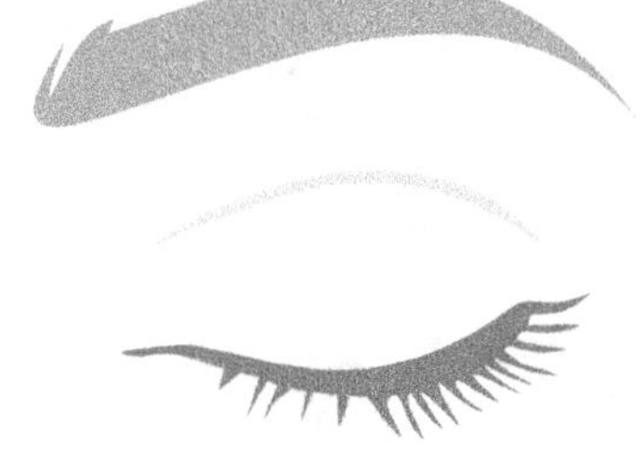
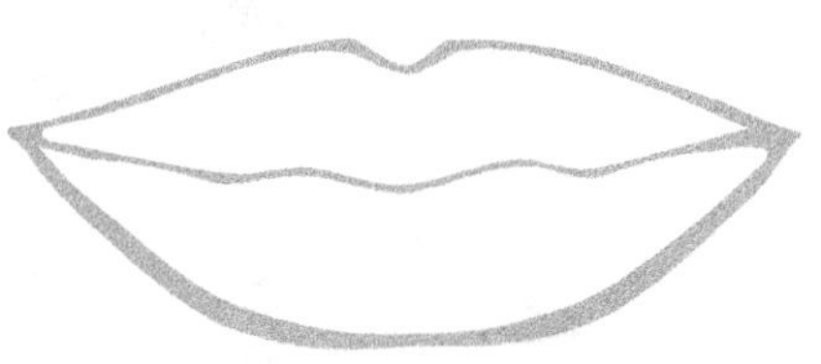

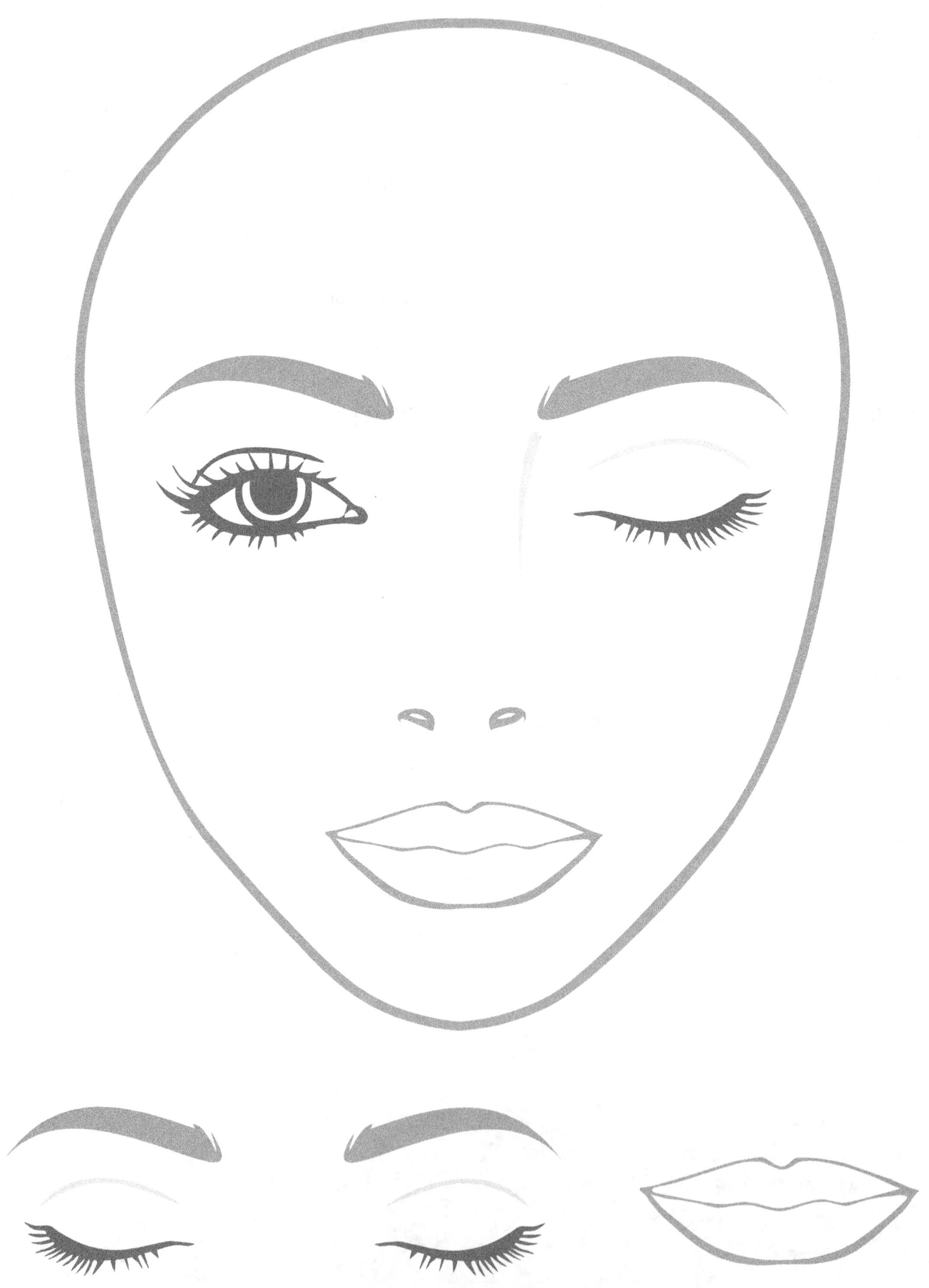

LOOK NAME _______________________   **FOR:** _______________________

◯ Daytime   ◯ Evening

FACE

Moisturizer

____

Primer

____

Powder

____

Highlight/Blush

____

Concealer

____

Foundation

____

Contour

____

EYES

Brows

____

Eyelid

____

Liner

____

Crease

____

Mascara

____

LIPS

Liner

____

Lip Color

____

Gloss

____

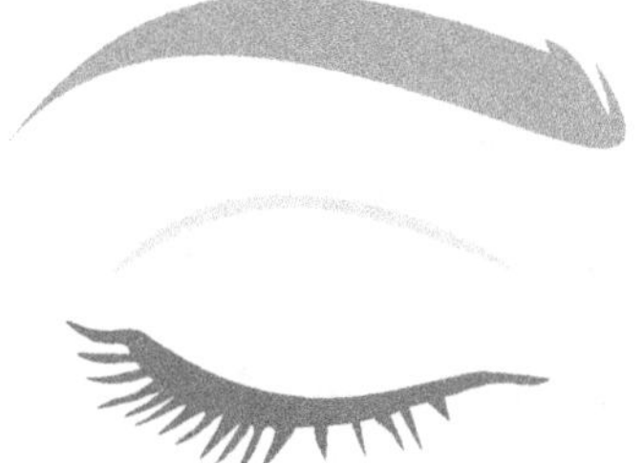
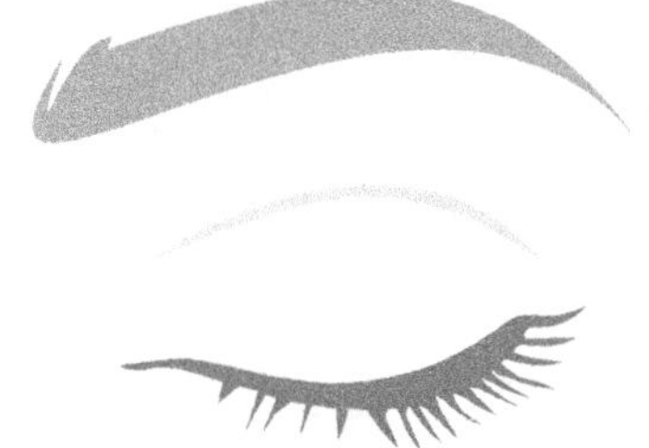
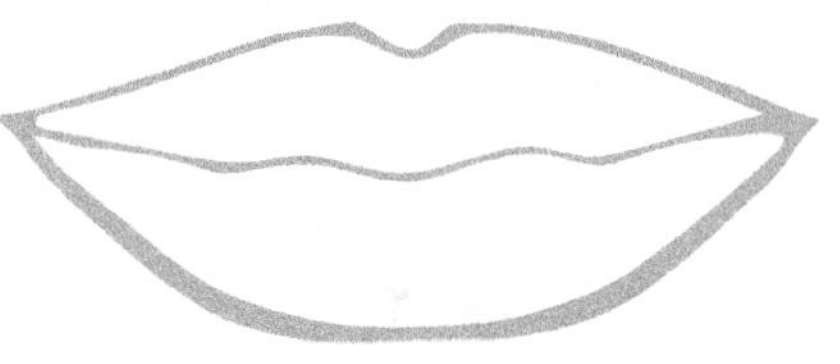

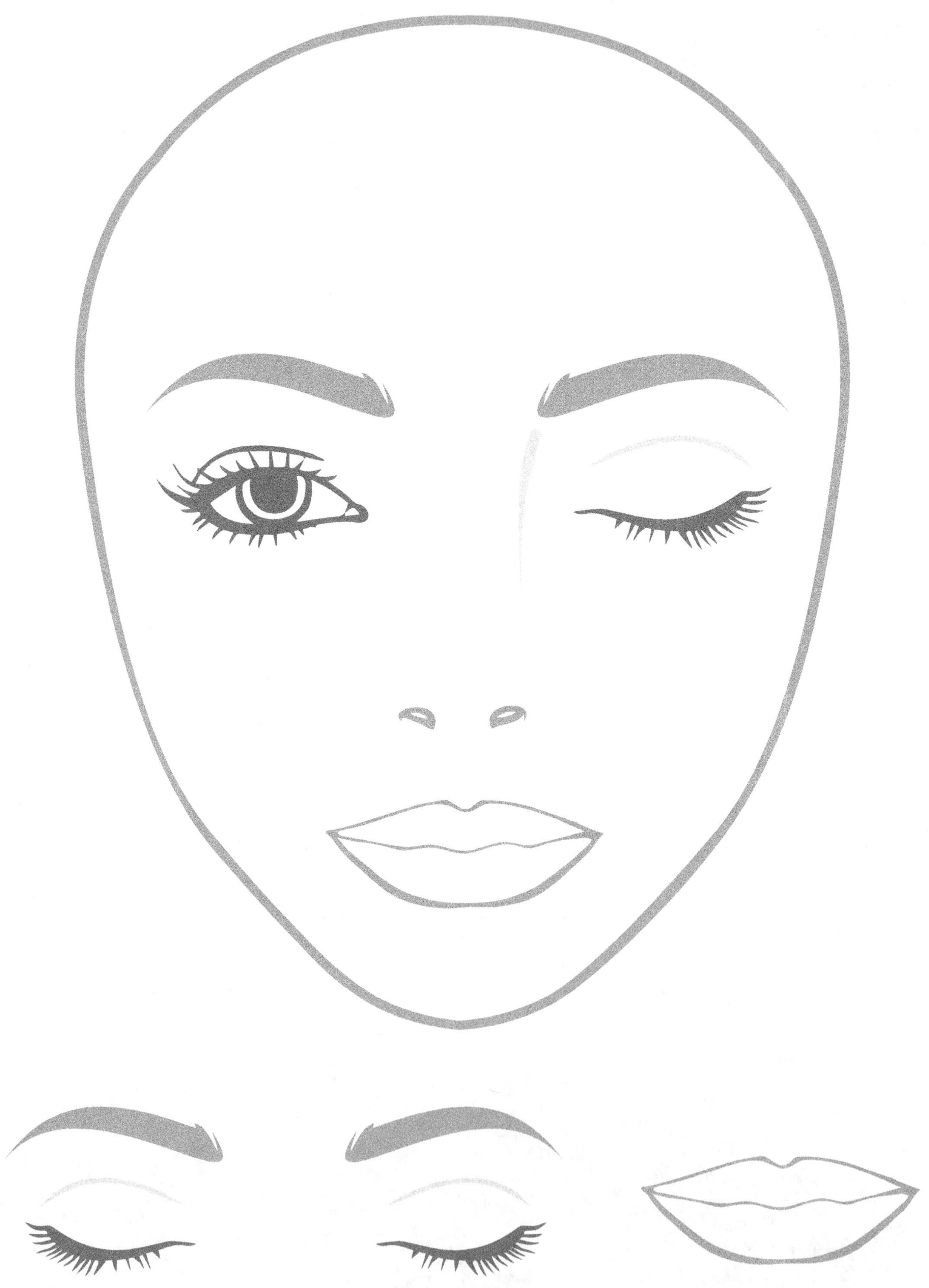

LOOK NAME ___________________   FOR: ___________________

○ Daytime   ○ Evening

FACE

Moisturizer

____

Primer

____

Powder

____

Highlight/Blush

____

Concealer

____

Foundation

____

Contour

____

EYES

Brows

____

Eyelid

____

Liner

____

Crease

____

Mascara

LIPS

Liner

____

Lip Color

____

Gloss

____

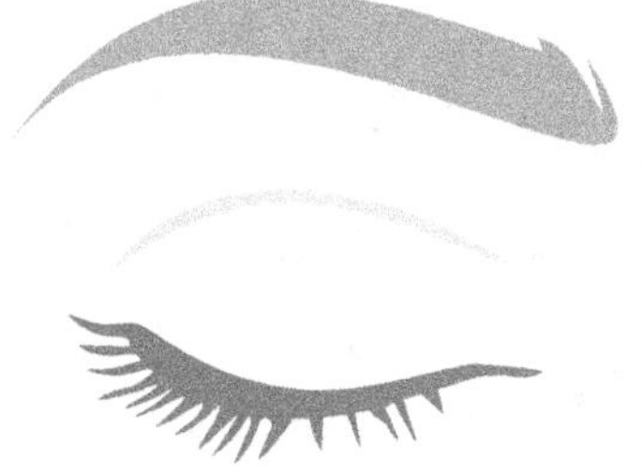

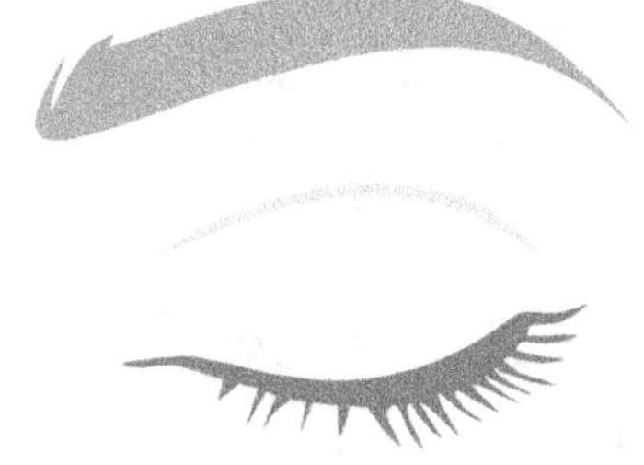

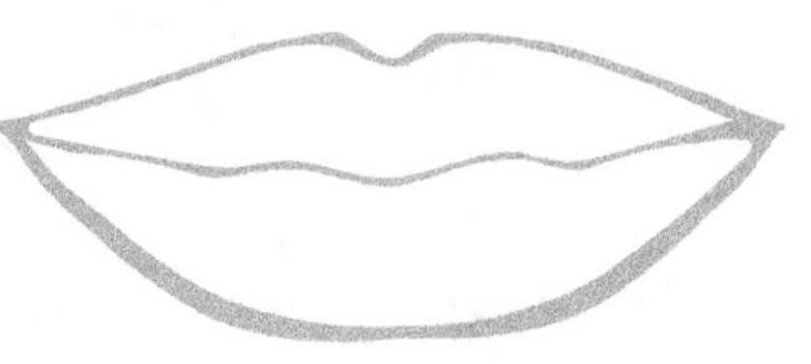

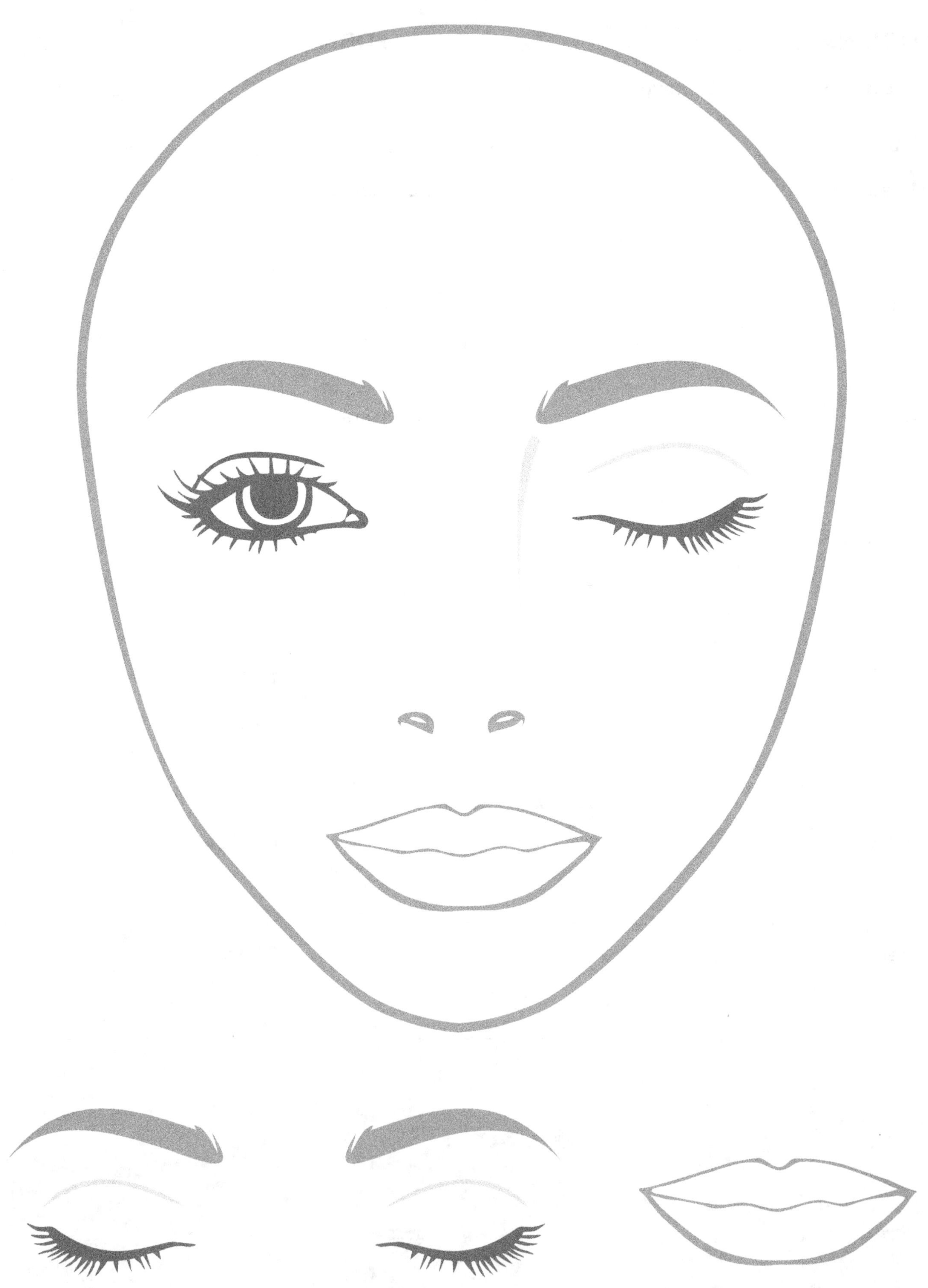

LOOK NAME __________________   **FOR:** __________________

◯ Daytime   ◯ Evening

FACE

Moisturizer

____

Primer

____

Powder

____

Highlight/Blush

____

Concealer

____

Foundation

____

Contour

____

EYES

Brows

____

Eyelid

____

Liner

____

Crease

____

Mascara

____

LIPS

Liner

____

Lip Color

____

Gloss

____

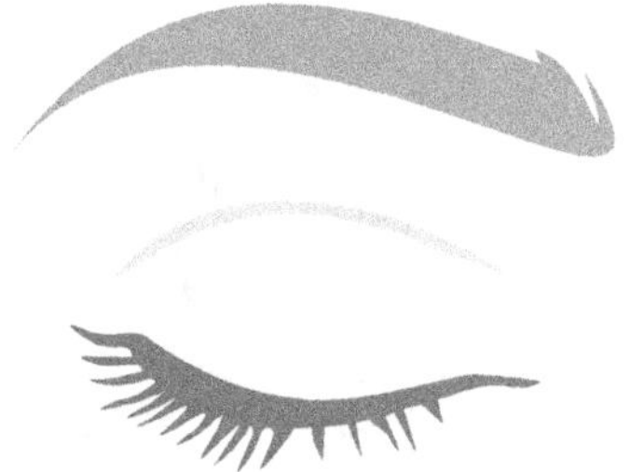
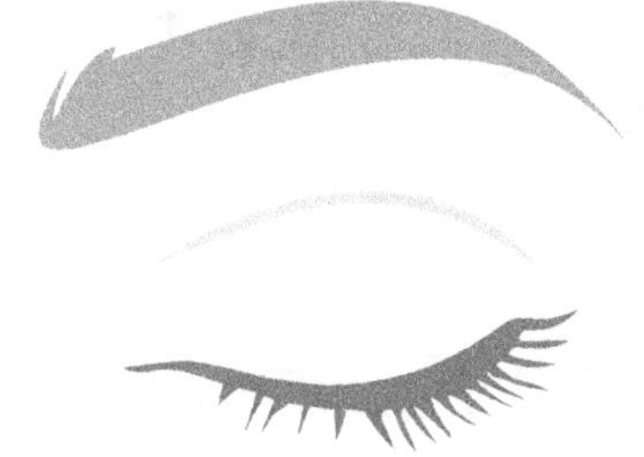
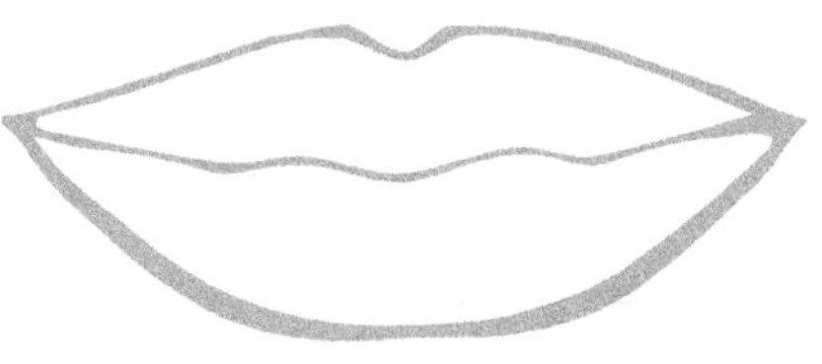

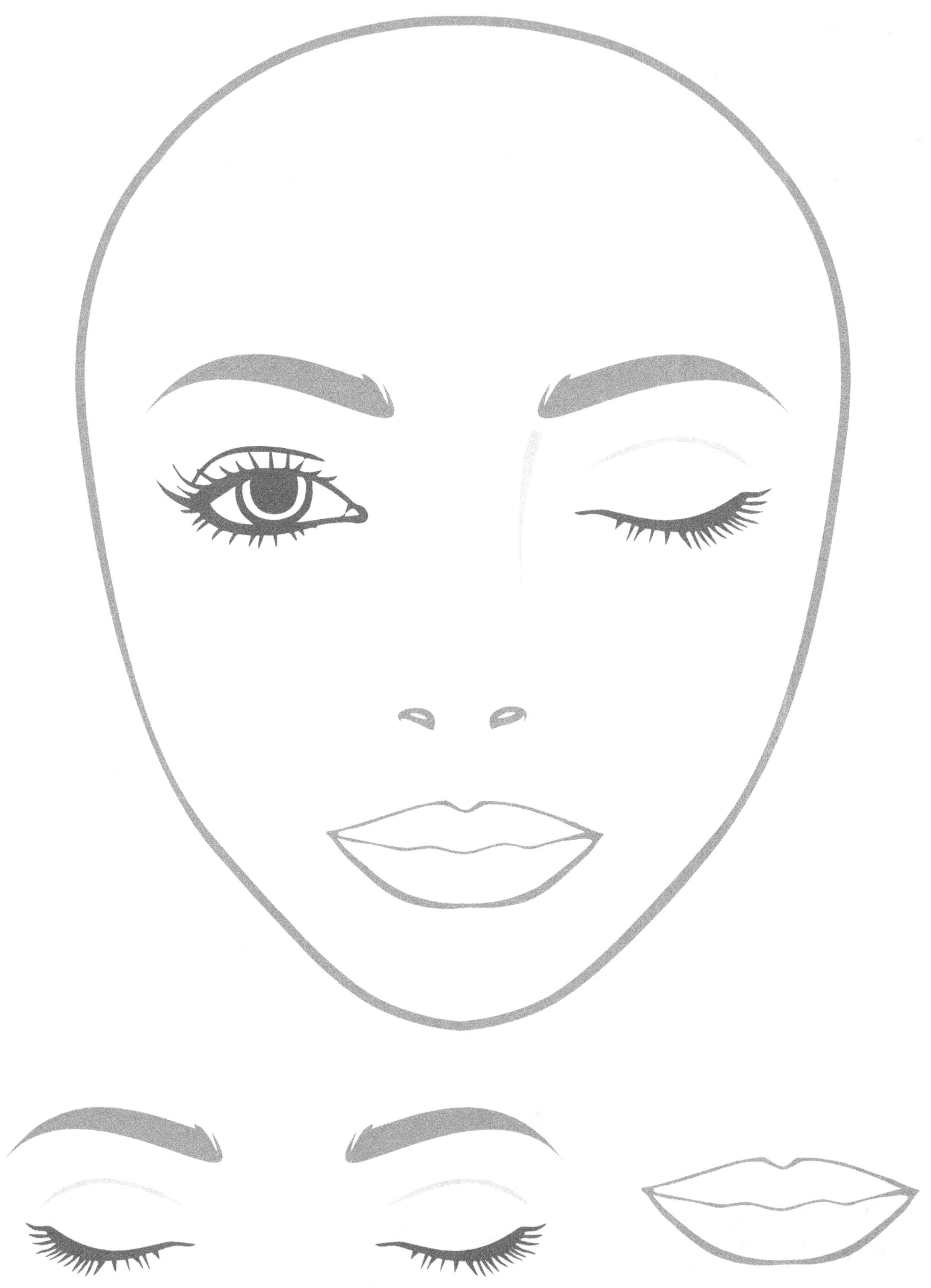

LOOK NAME ________________________ FOR: ________________________

◯ Daytime   ◯ Evening

FACE

Moisturizer

Concealer

Primer

Foundation

Powder

Contour

Highlight/Blush

EYES

Brows

Crease

Eyelid

Mascara

Liner

LIPS

Liner

Lip Color

Gloss

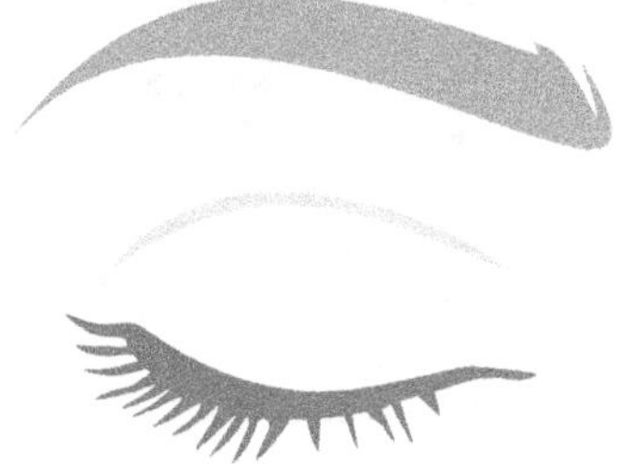
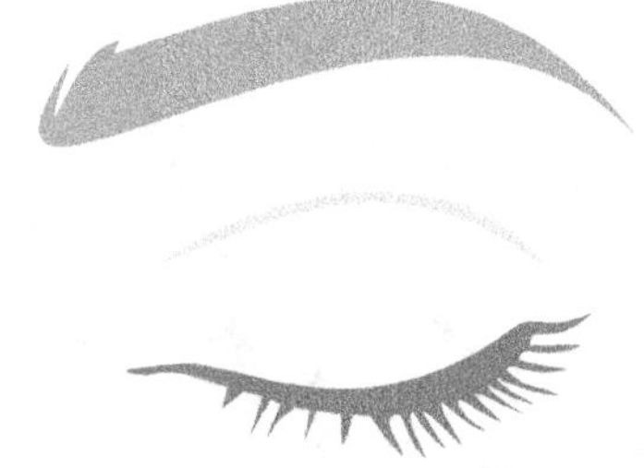
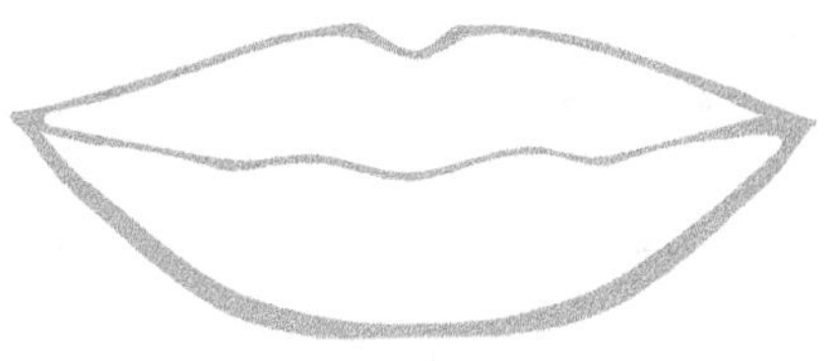

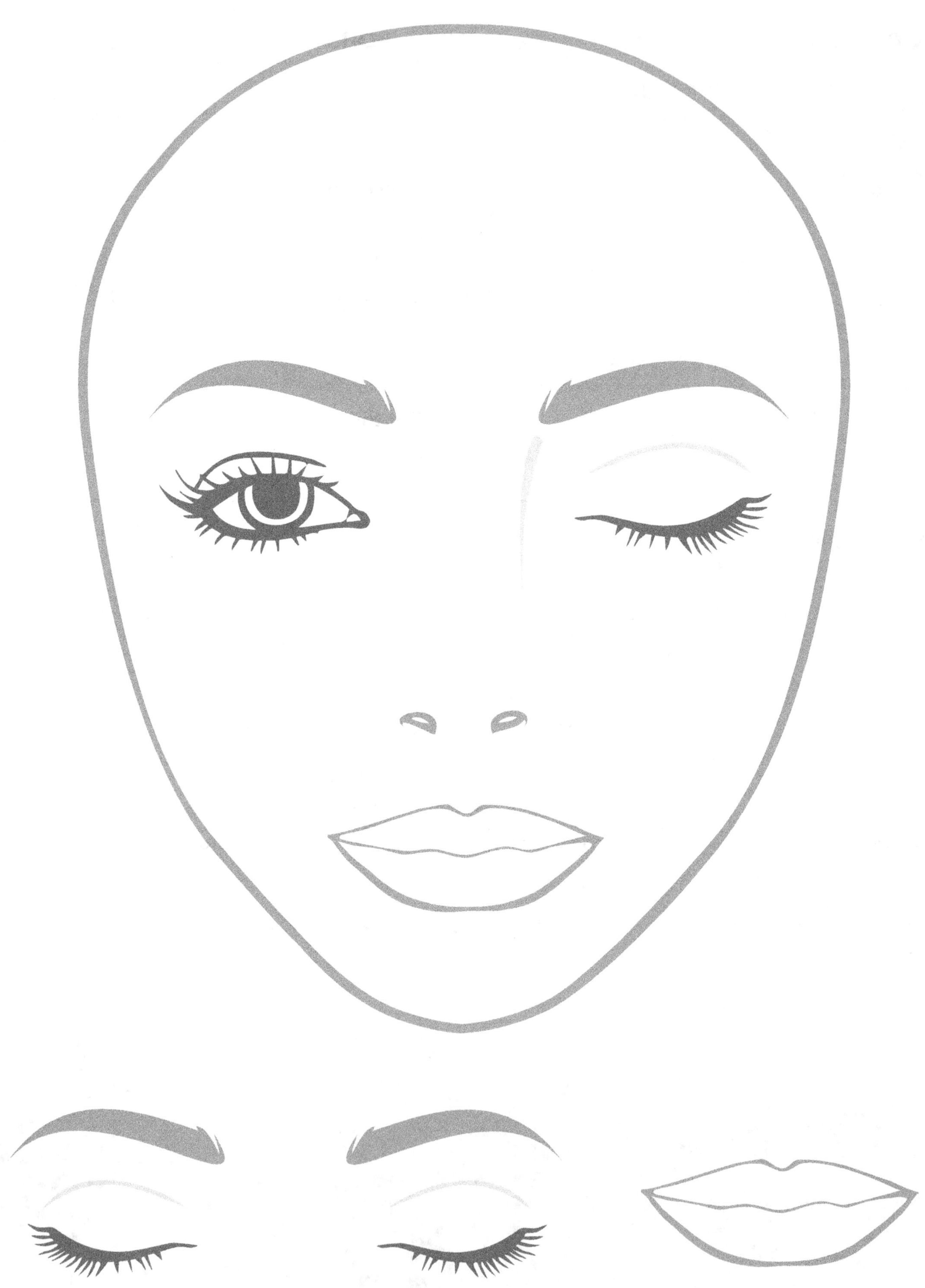

LOOK NAME _______________________   **FOR:** _______________________

○ Daytime   ○ Evening

FACE

Moisturizer

____

Primer

____

Powder

____

Highlight/Blush

____

Concealer

____

Foundation

____

Contour

____

EYES

Brows

____

Eyelid

____

Liner

____

Crease

____

Mascara

____

LIPS

Liner

____

Lip Color

____

Gloss

____

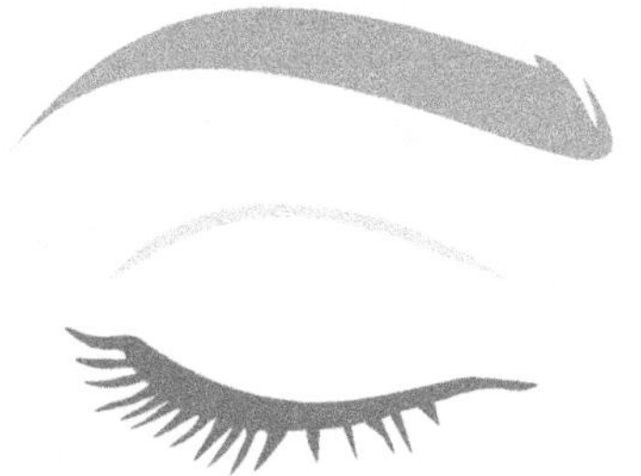
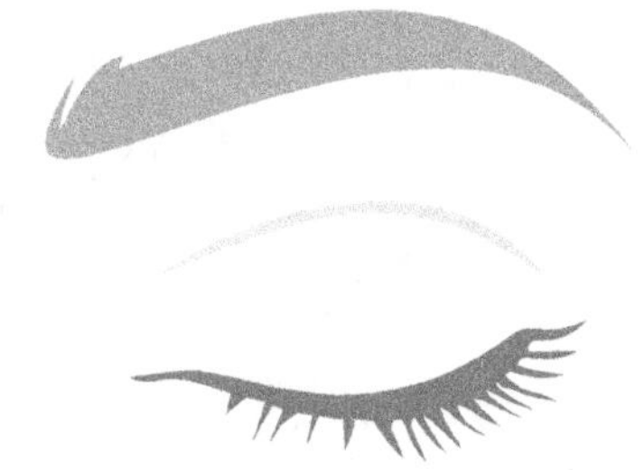
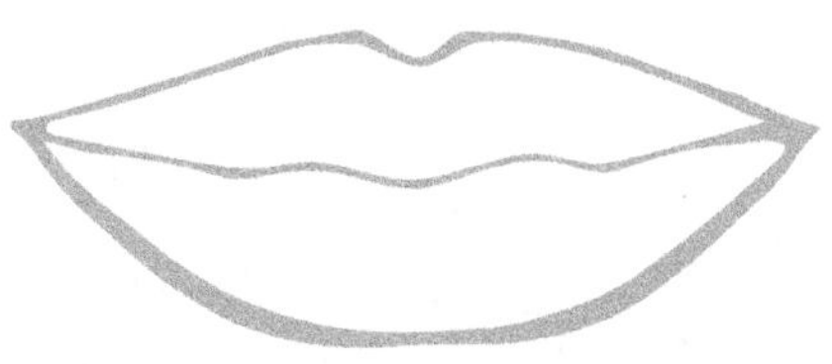

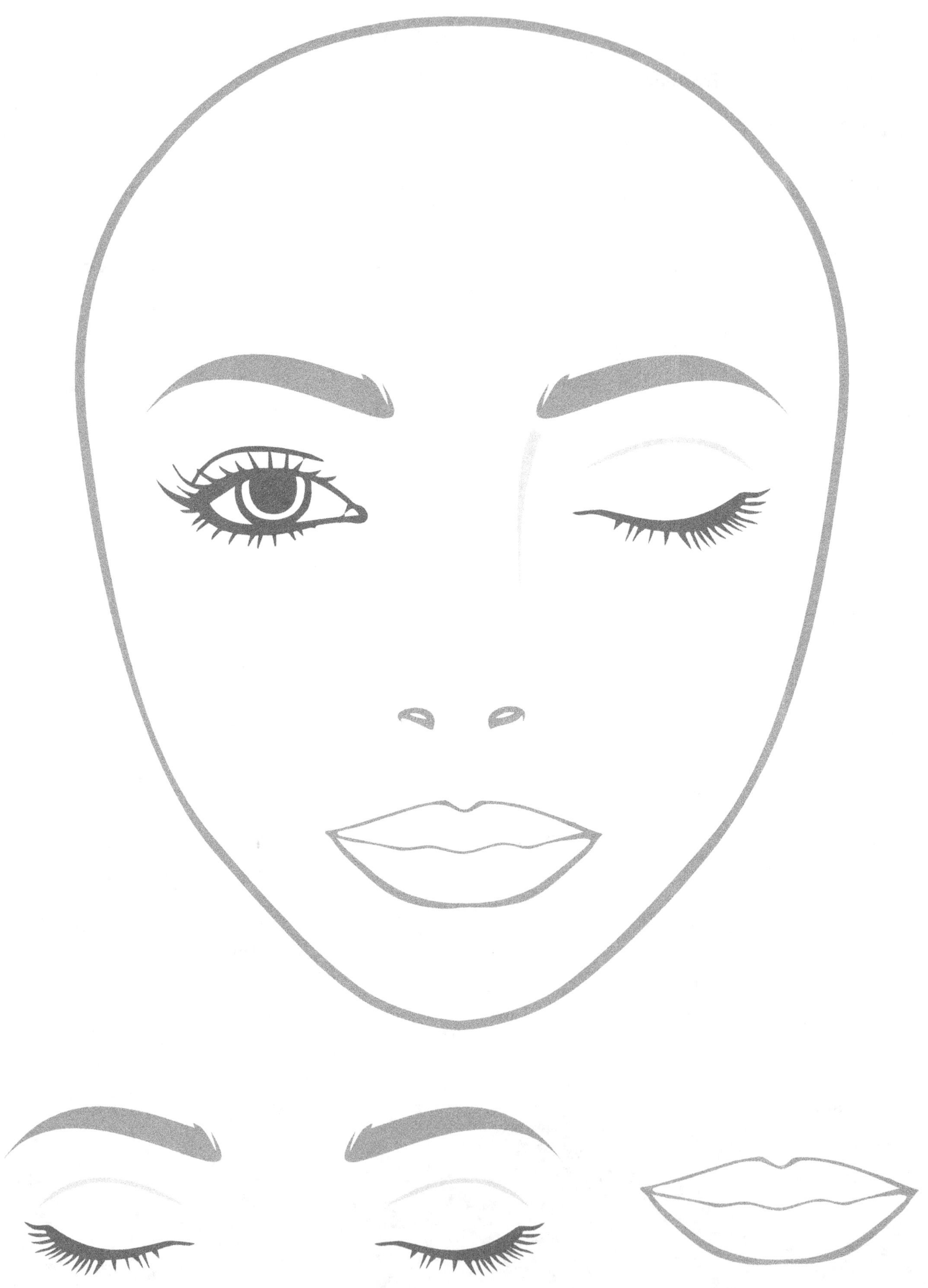

LOOK NAME _______________________   FOR: _______________________

○ Daytime   ○ Evening

FACE

Moisturizer

____

Primer

____

Powder

____

Highlight/Blush

____

Concealer

____

Foundation

____

Contour

____

EYES

Brows

____

Eyelid

____

Liner

____

Crease

____

Mascara

____

LIPS

Liner

____

Lip Color

____

Gloss

____

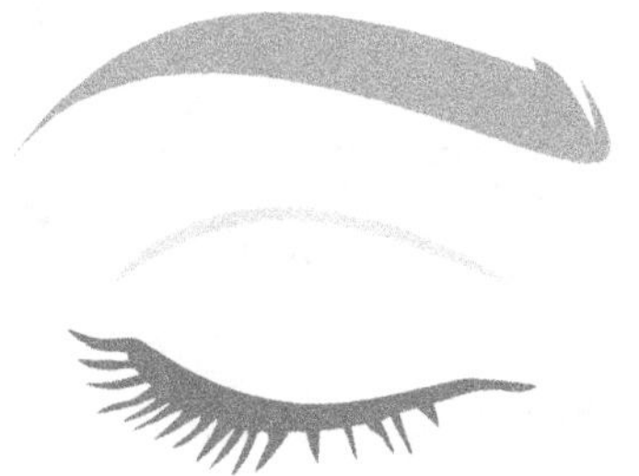

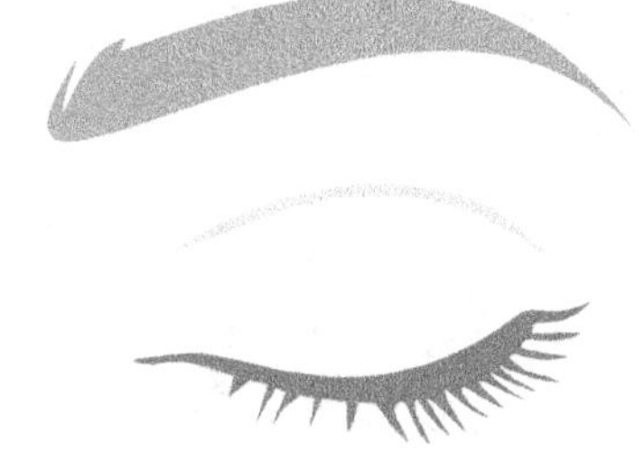

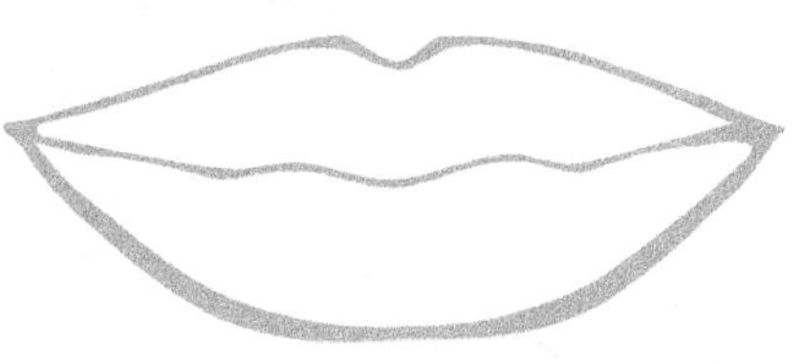

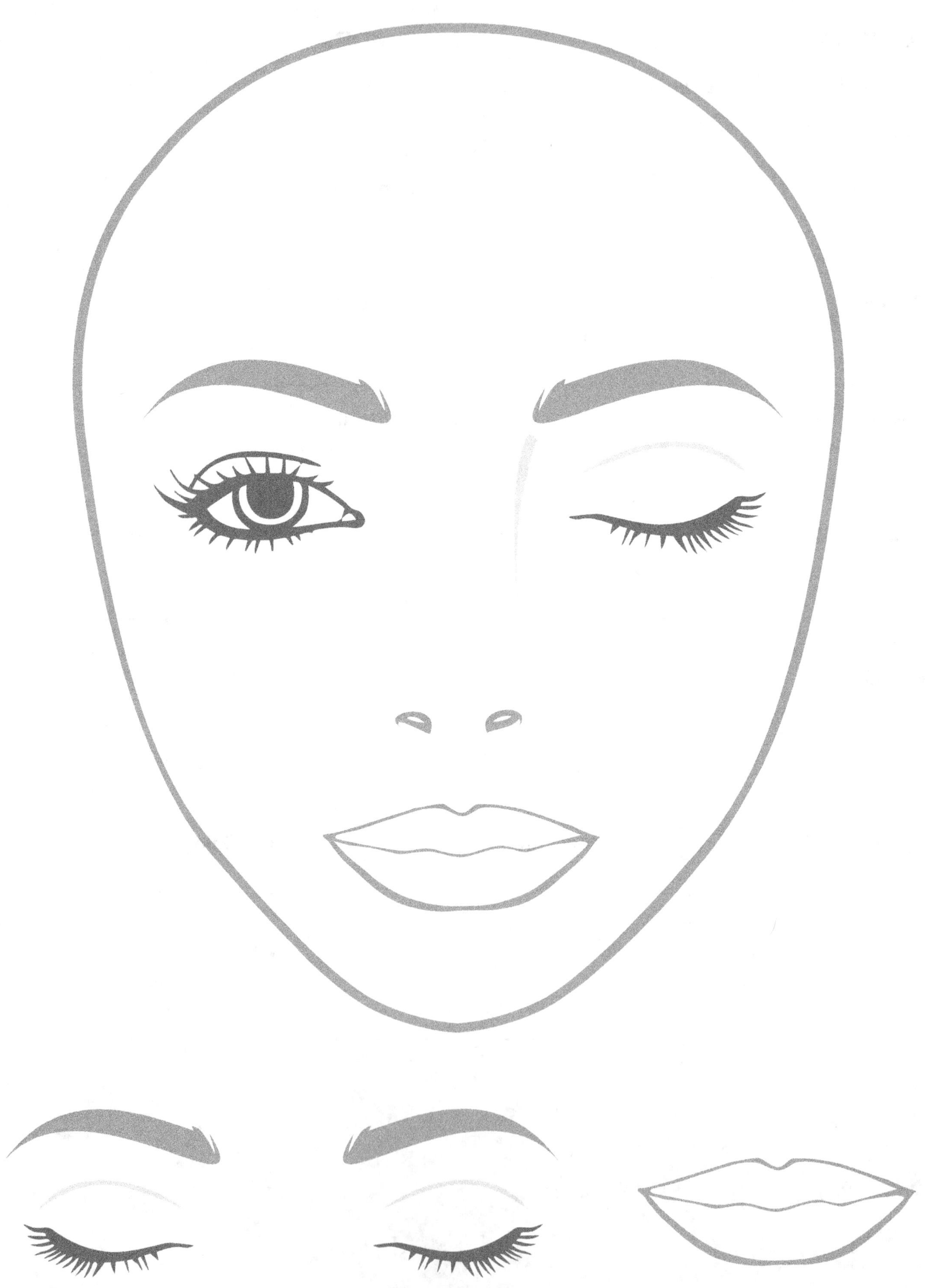

LOOK NAME ______________________   FOR: ______________________

◯ Daytime   ◯ Evening

FACE

Moisturizer

____

Primer

____

Powder

____

Highlight/Blush

____

Concealer

____

Foundation

____

Contour

____

EYES

Brows	Crease	
Eyelid	Mascara	
Liner		

LIPS

Liner

____

Lip Color

____

Gloss

____

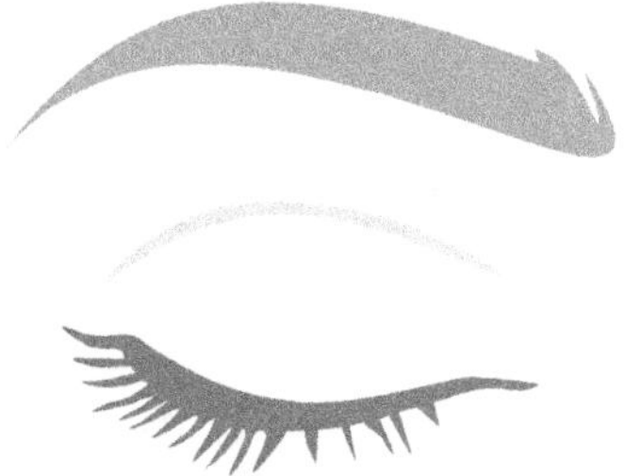
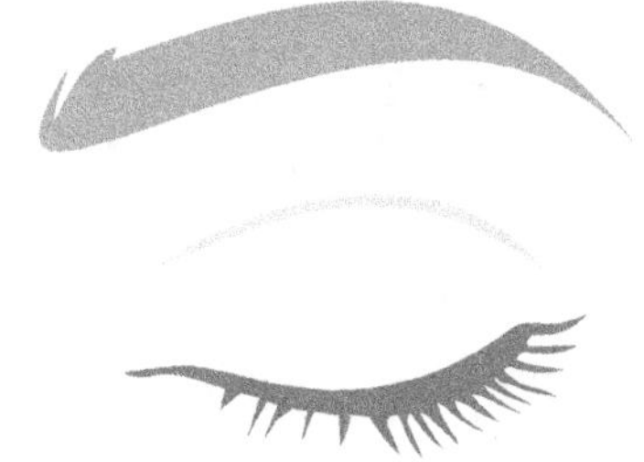
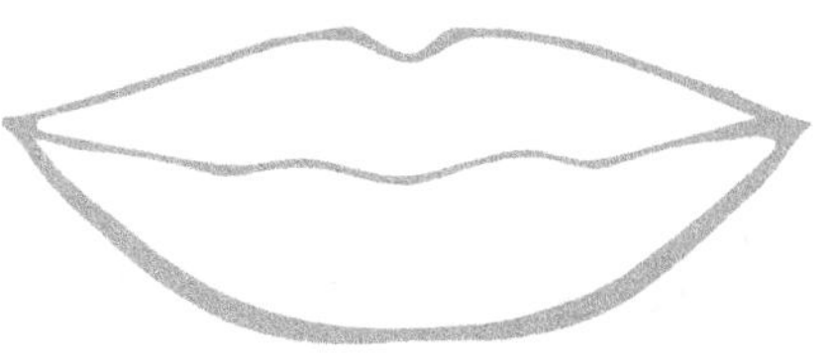

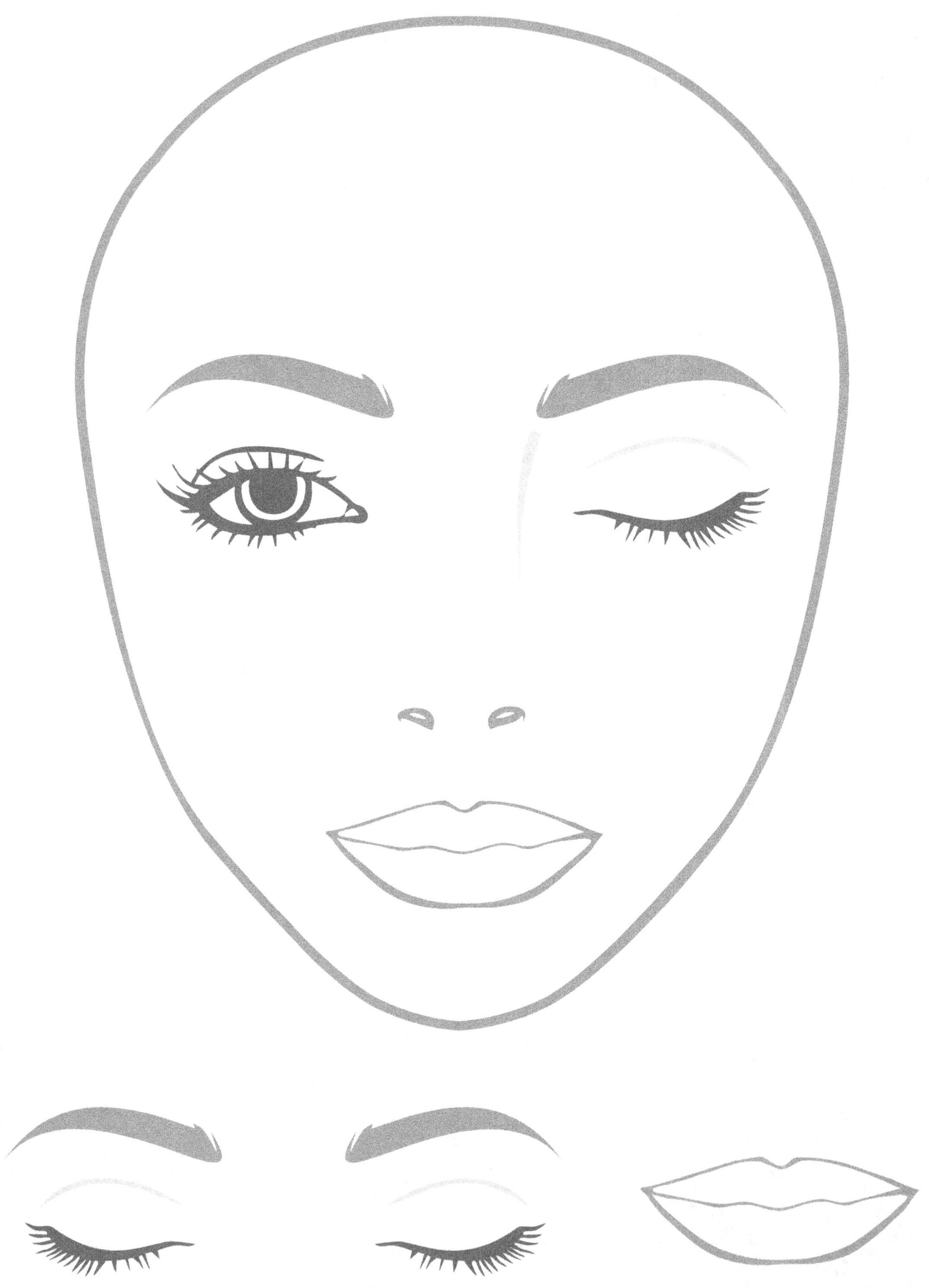

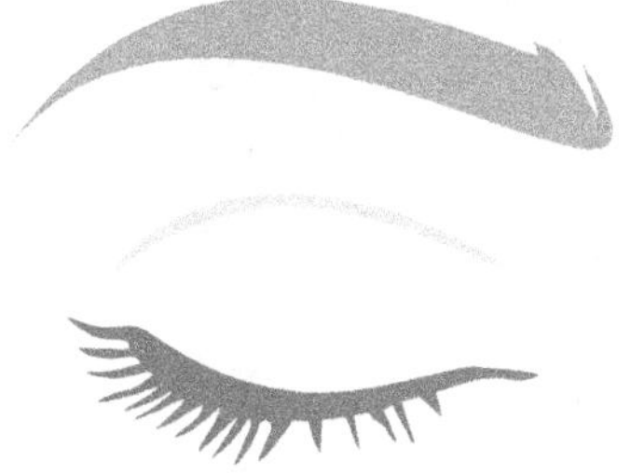
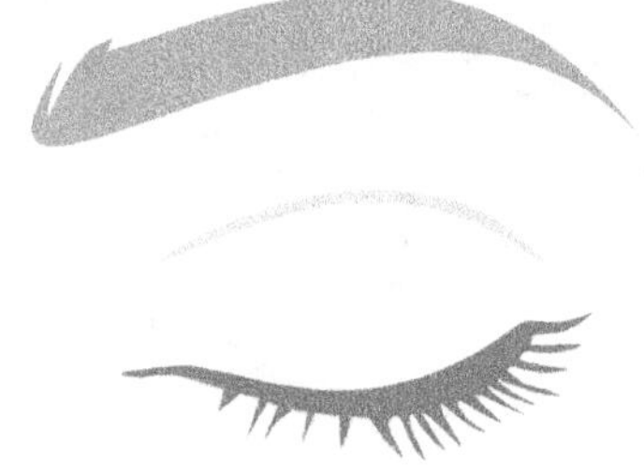
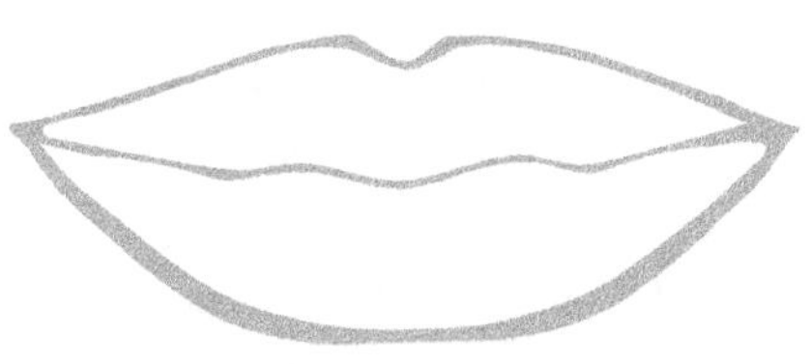

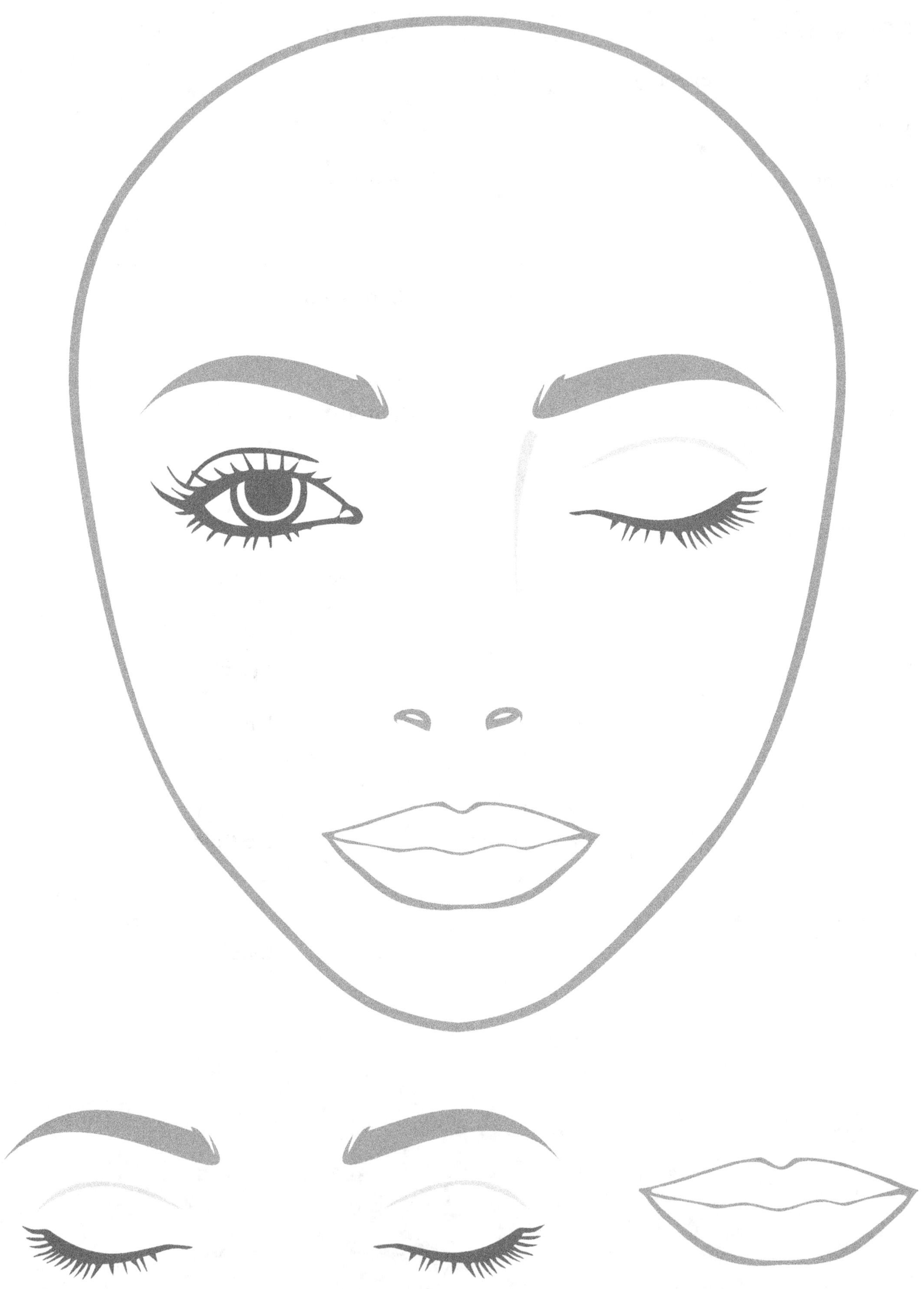

LOOK NAME ________________________ **FOR:** ________________________

◯ Daytime   ◯ Evening

FACE

Moisturizer

____

Primer

____

Powder

____

Highlight/Blush

____

Concealer

____

Foundation

____

Contour

____

EYES

Brows

____

Eyelid

____

Liner

____

Crease

____

Mascara

____

LIPS

Liner

____

Lip Color

____

Gloss

____

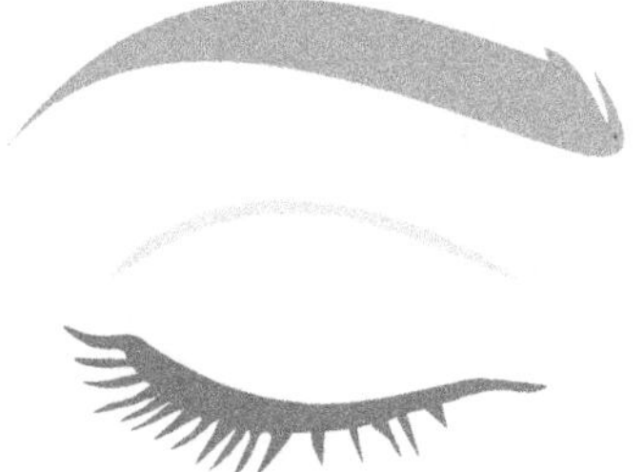

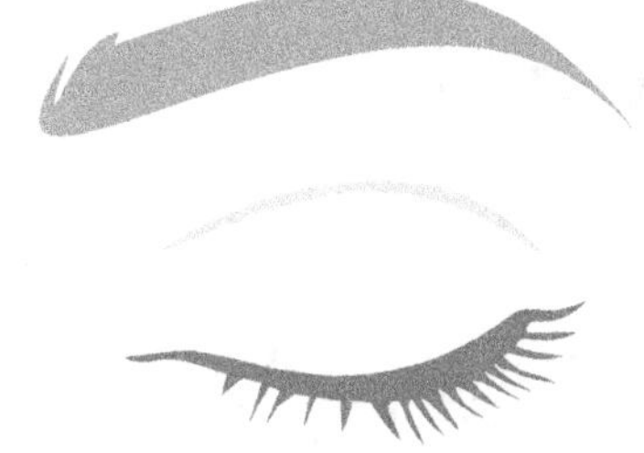

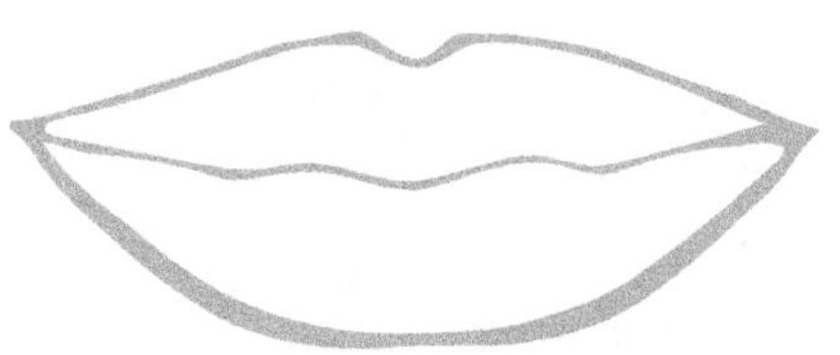

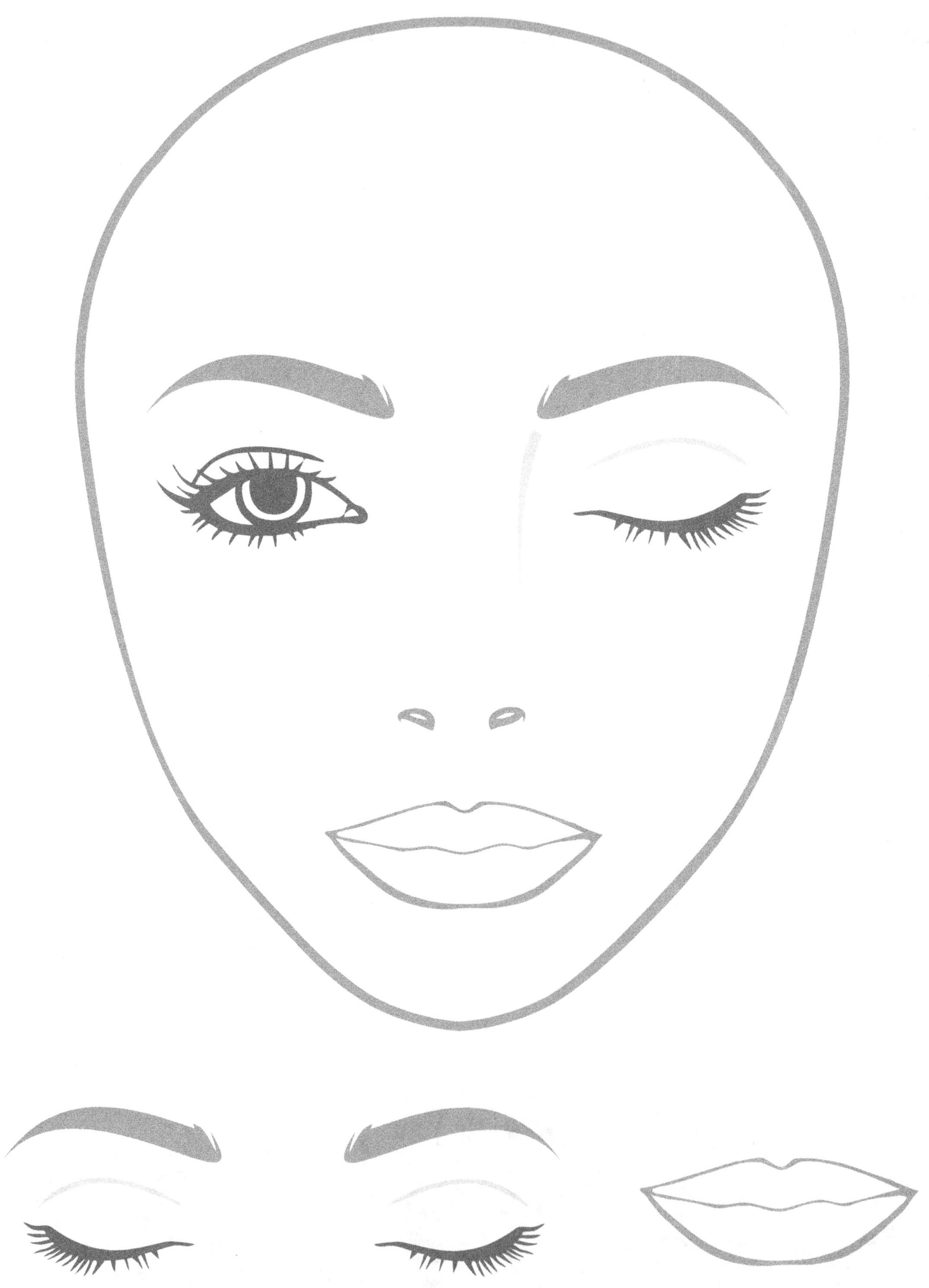

LOOK NAME _______________________   FOR: _______________________

○ Daytime   ○ Evening

FACE

Moisturizer

____

Primer

____

Powder

____

Highlight/Blush

____

Concealer

____

Foundation

____

Contour

____

EYES

Brows

____

Eyelid

____

Liner

____

Crease

____

Mascara

____

LIPS

Liner

____

Lip Color

____

Gloss

____

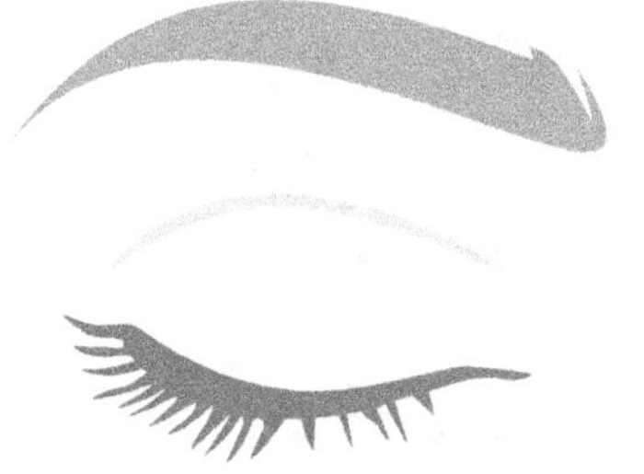
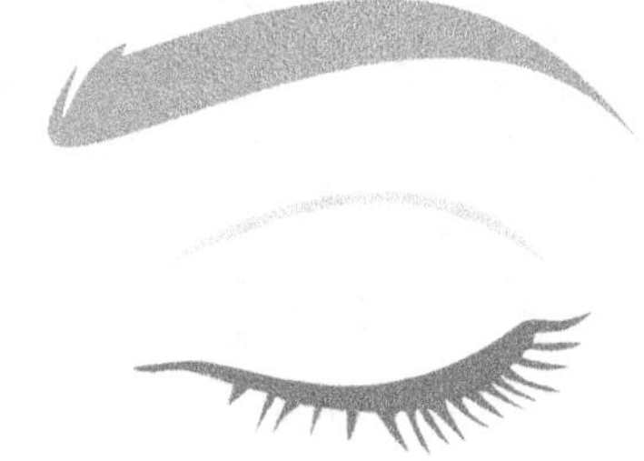
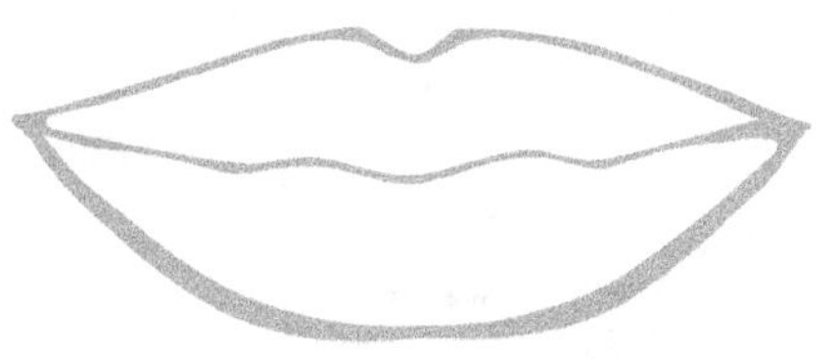

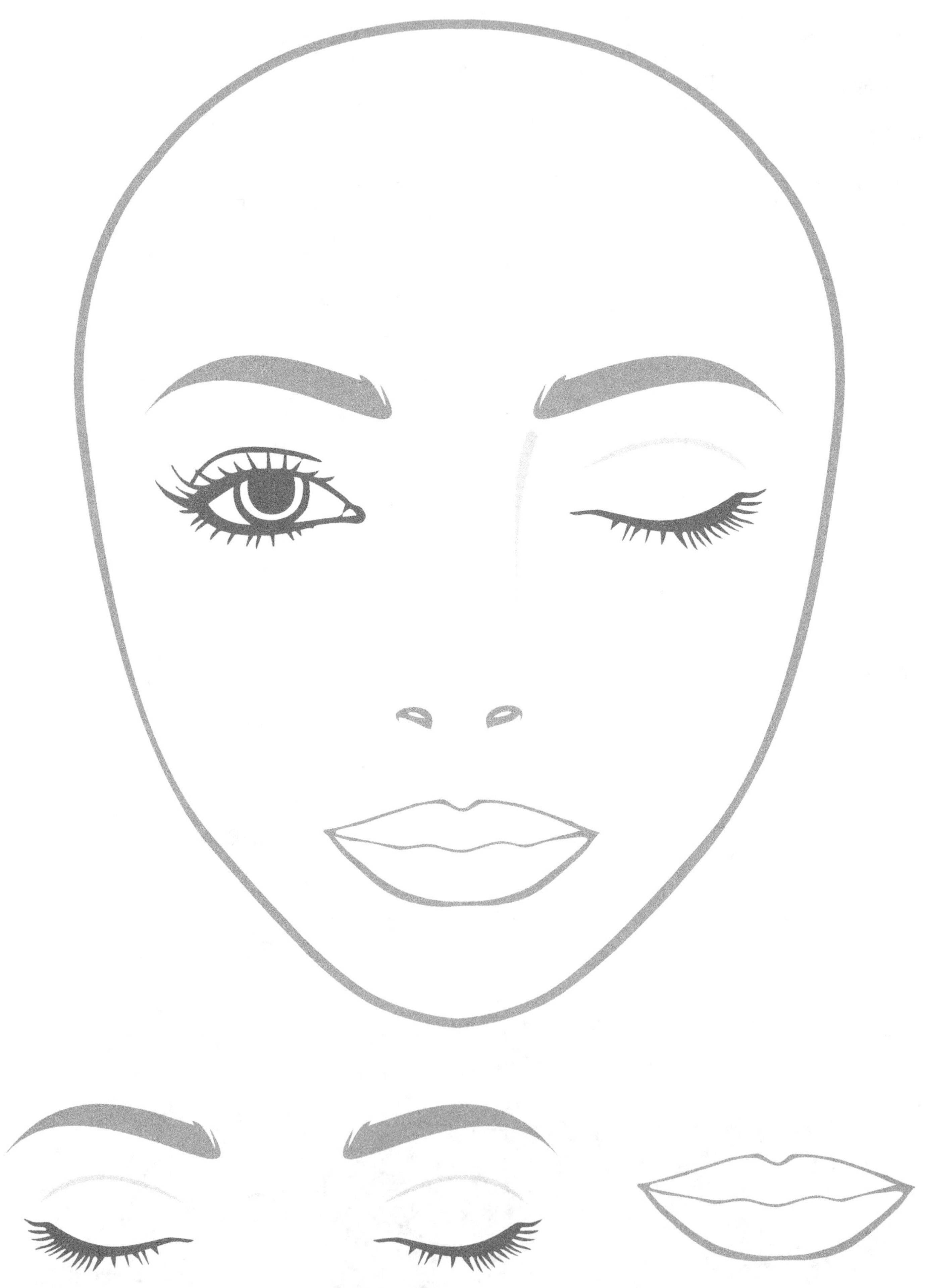

LOOK NAME _______________________   FOR: _______________________

○ Daytime   ○ Evening

FACE

Moisturizer

____

Primer

____

Powder

____

Highlight/Blush

____

Concealer

____

Foundation

____

Contour

____

EYES

Brows

____

Eyelid

____

Liner

____

Crease

____

Mascara

____

LIPS

Liner

____

Lip Color

____

Gloss

____

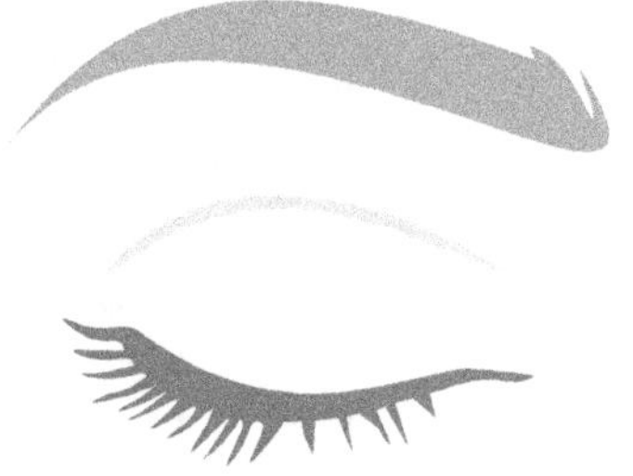
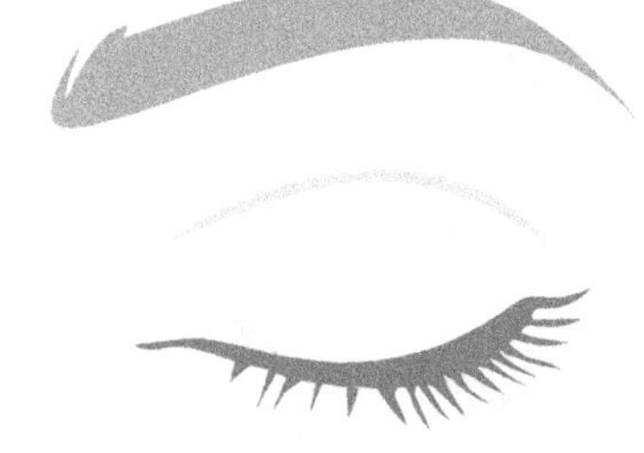
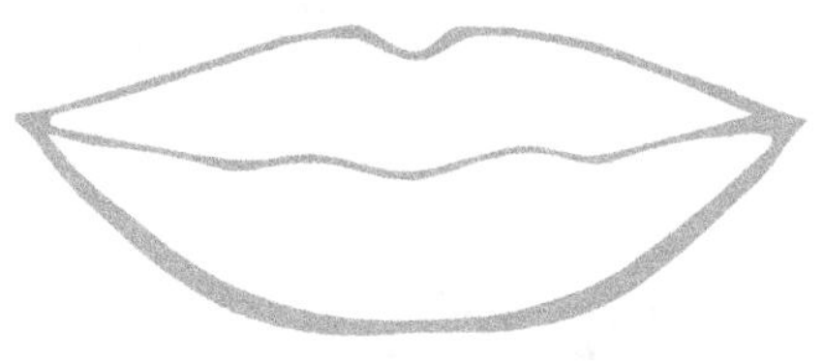

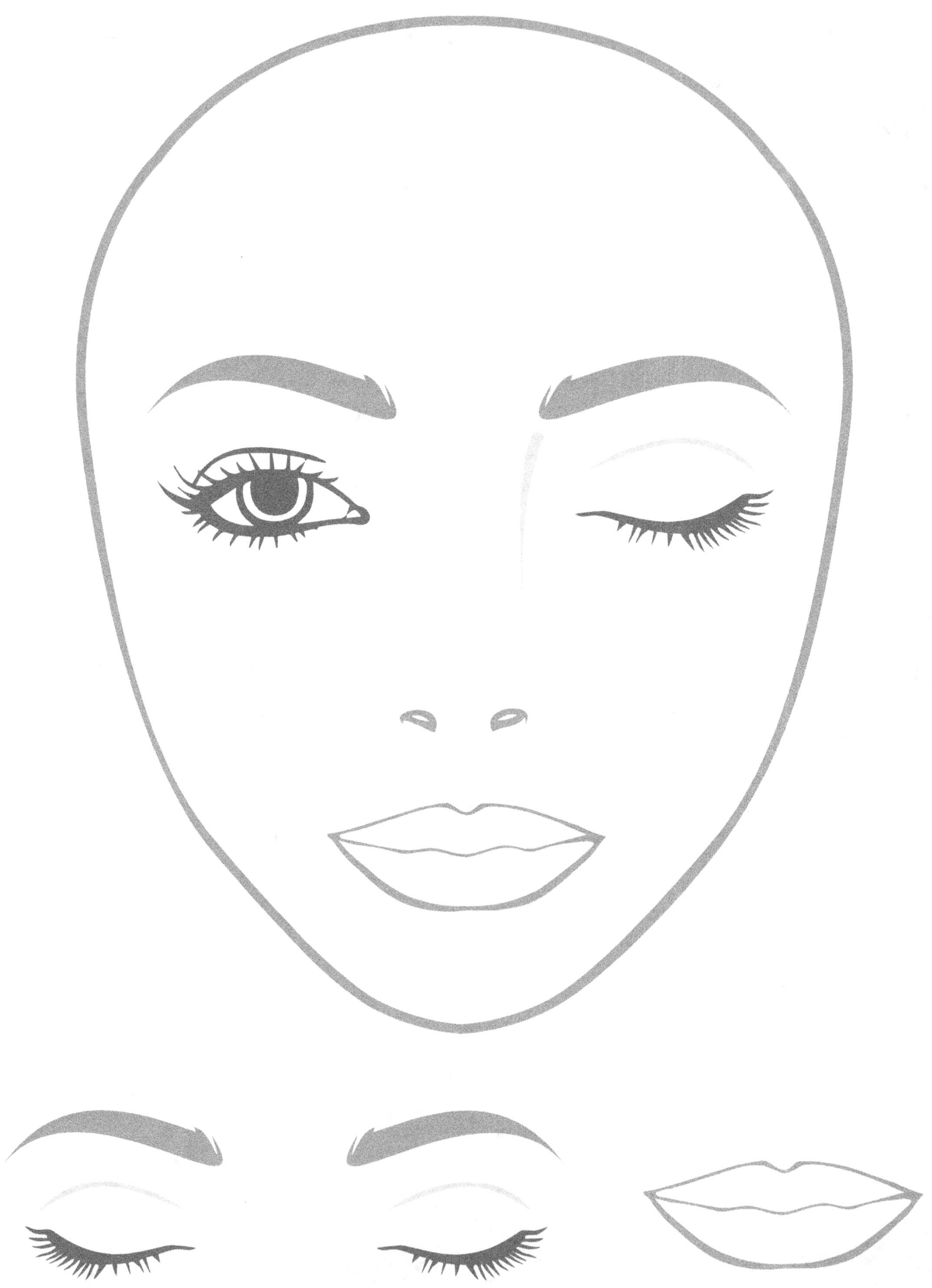

LOOK NAME __________________   FOR: __________________

◯ Daytime   ◯ Evening

FACE

Moisturizer

____

Primer

____

Powder

____

Highlight/Blush

____

Concealer

____

Foundation

____

Contour

____

EYES

Brows

____

Eyelid

____

Liner

Crease

____

Mascara

____

LIPS

Liner

____

Lip Color

____

Gloss

____

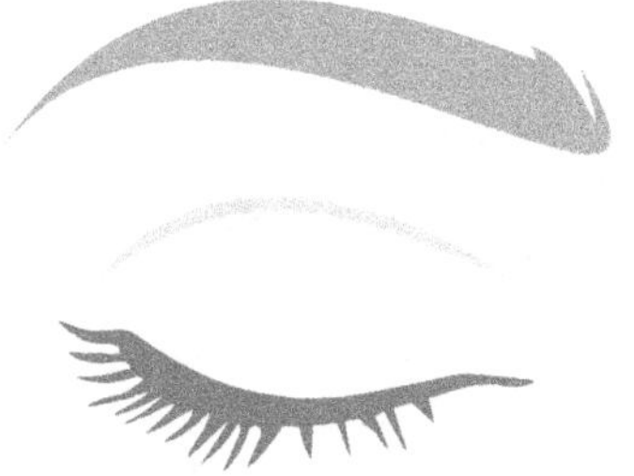
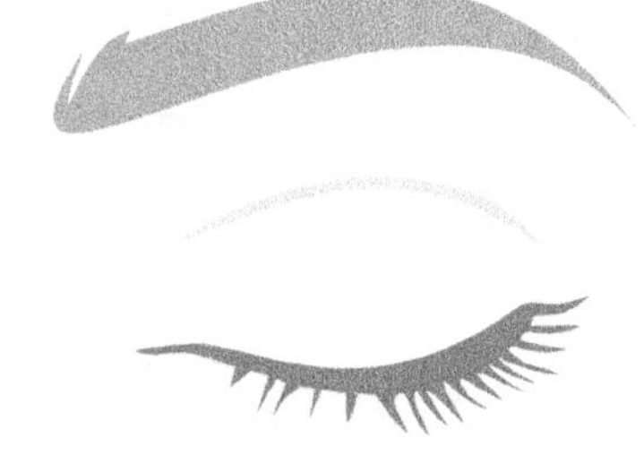
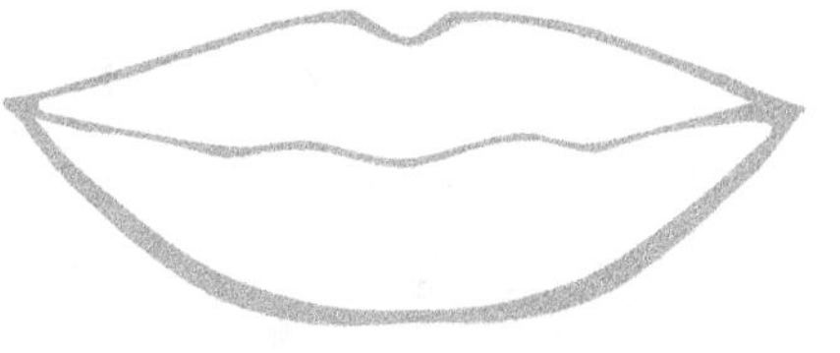

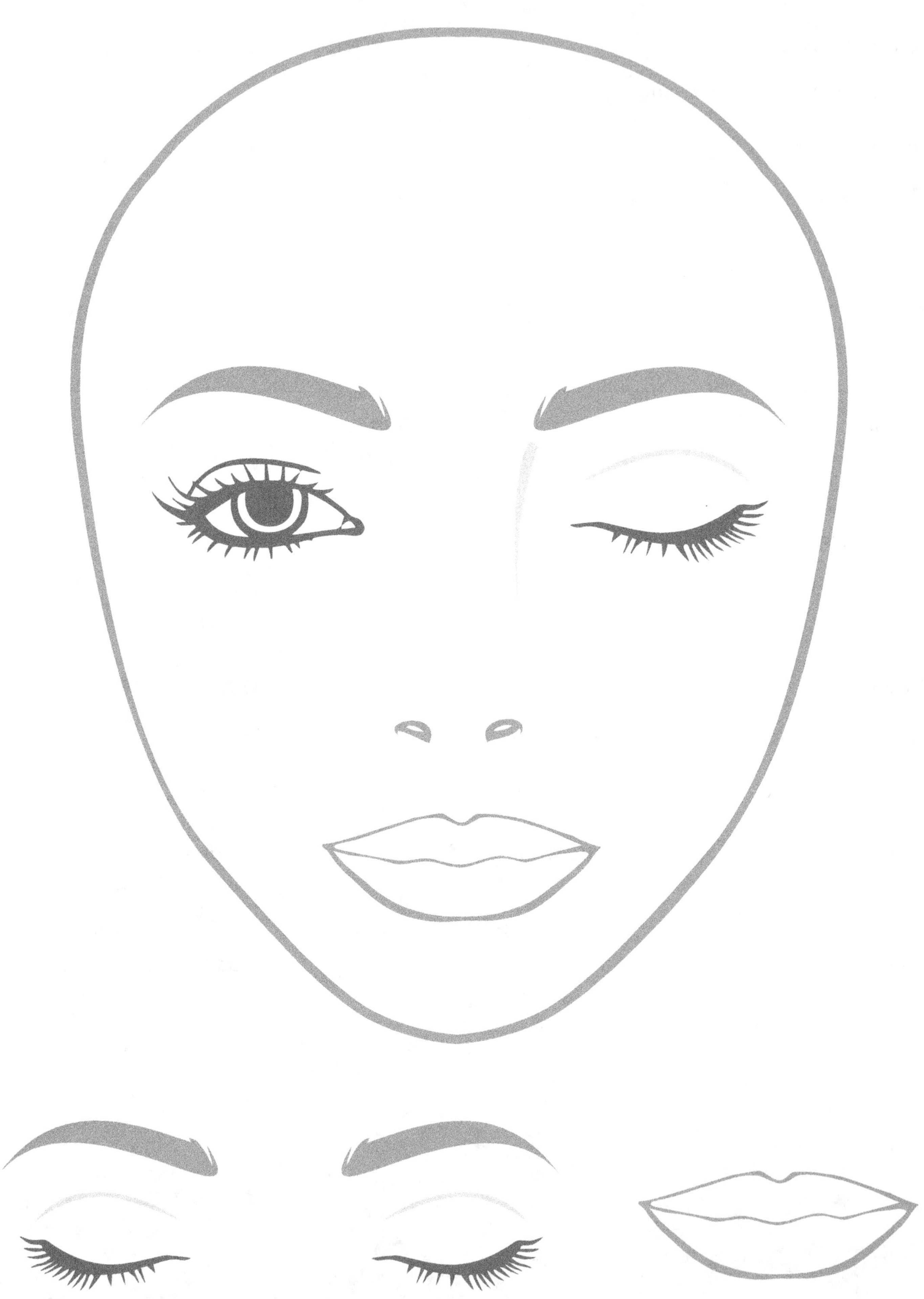

LOOK NAME ___________________ FOR: ___________________

○ Daytime   ○ Evening

FACE

Moisturizer

____

Primer

____

Powder

____

Highlight/Blush

____

Concealer

____

Foundation

____

Contour

____

EYES

Brows

____

Eyelid

____

Liner

____

Crease

____

Mascara

____

LIPS

Liner

____

Lip Color

____

Gloss

____

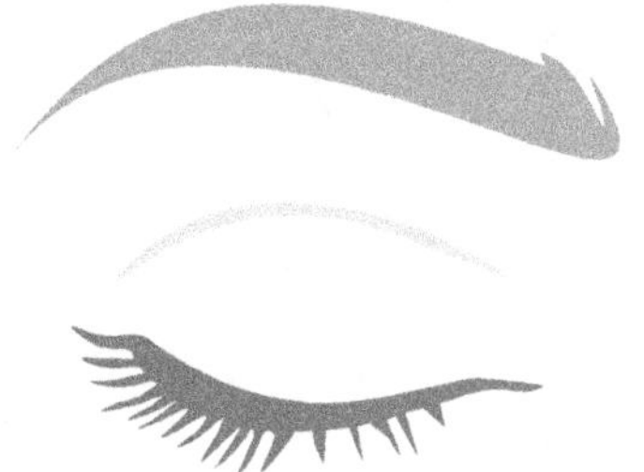
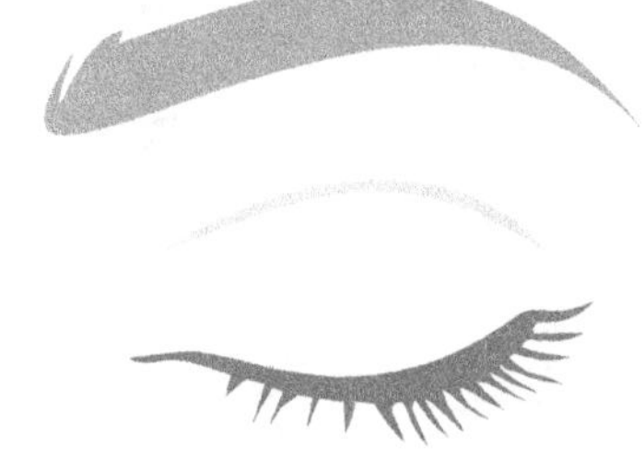
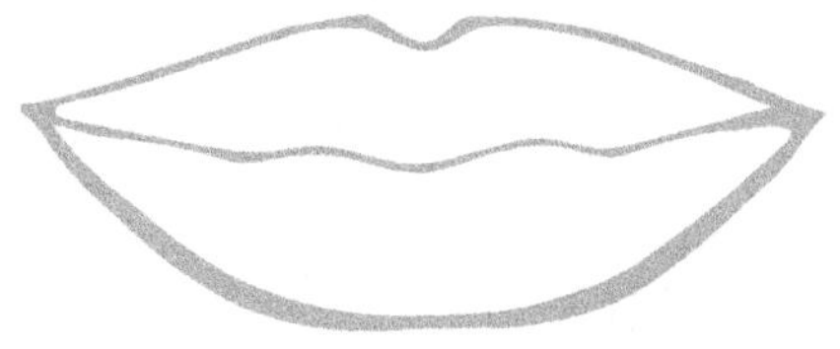

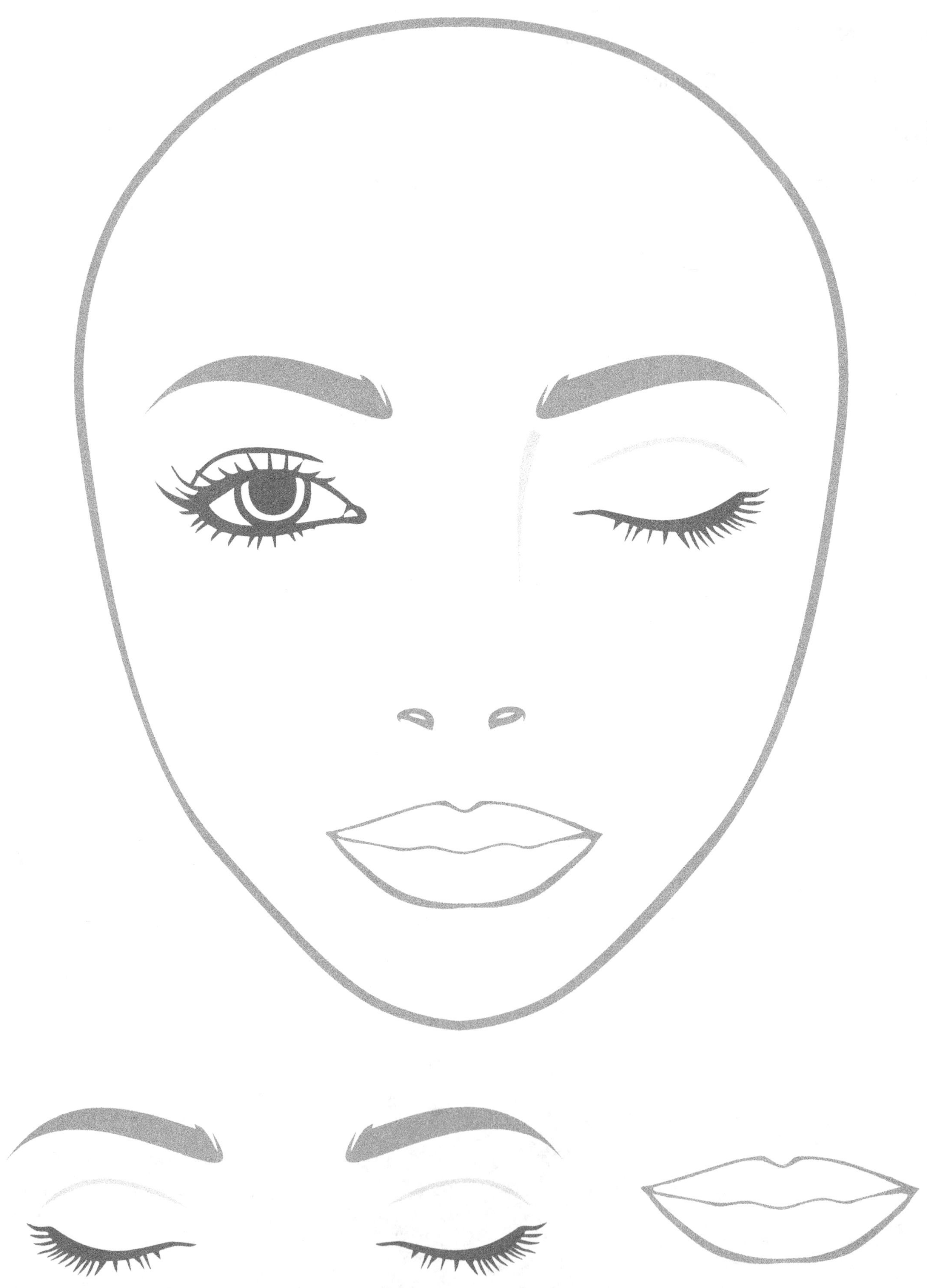

LOOK NAME ___________________________   FOR: ___________________________

◯ Daytime   ◯ Evening

FACE

Moisturizer
____

Primer
____

Powder
____

Highlight/Blush
____

Concealer
____

Foundation
____

Contour
____

EYES

Brows
____

Eyelid
____

Liner
____

Crease
____

Mascara
____

LIPS

Liner
____

Lip Color
____

Gloss
____

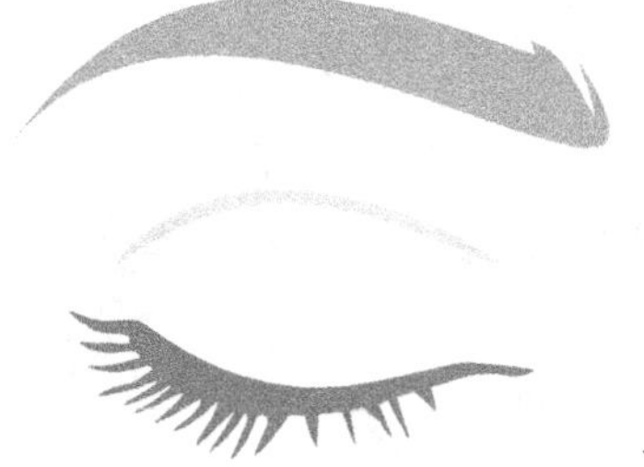
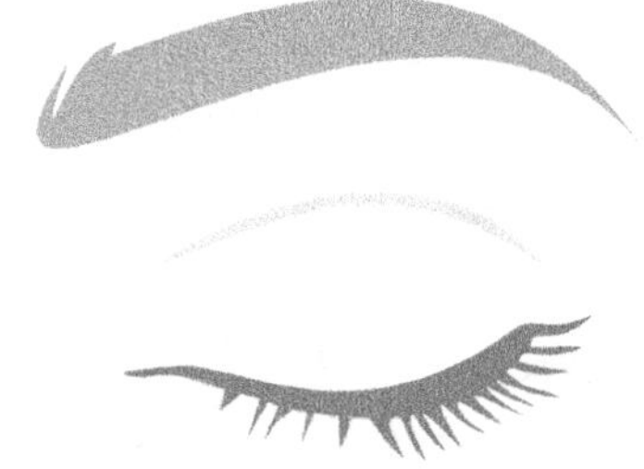
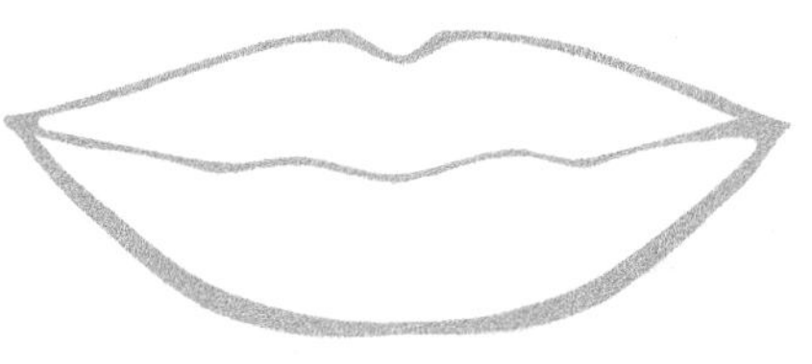

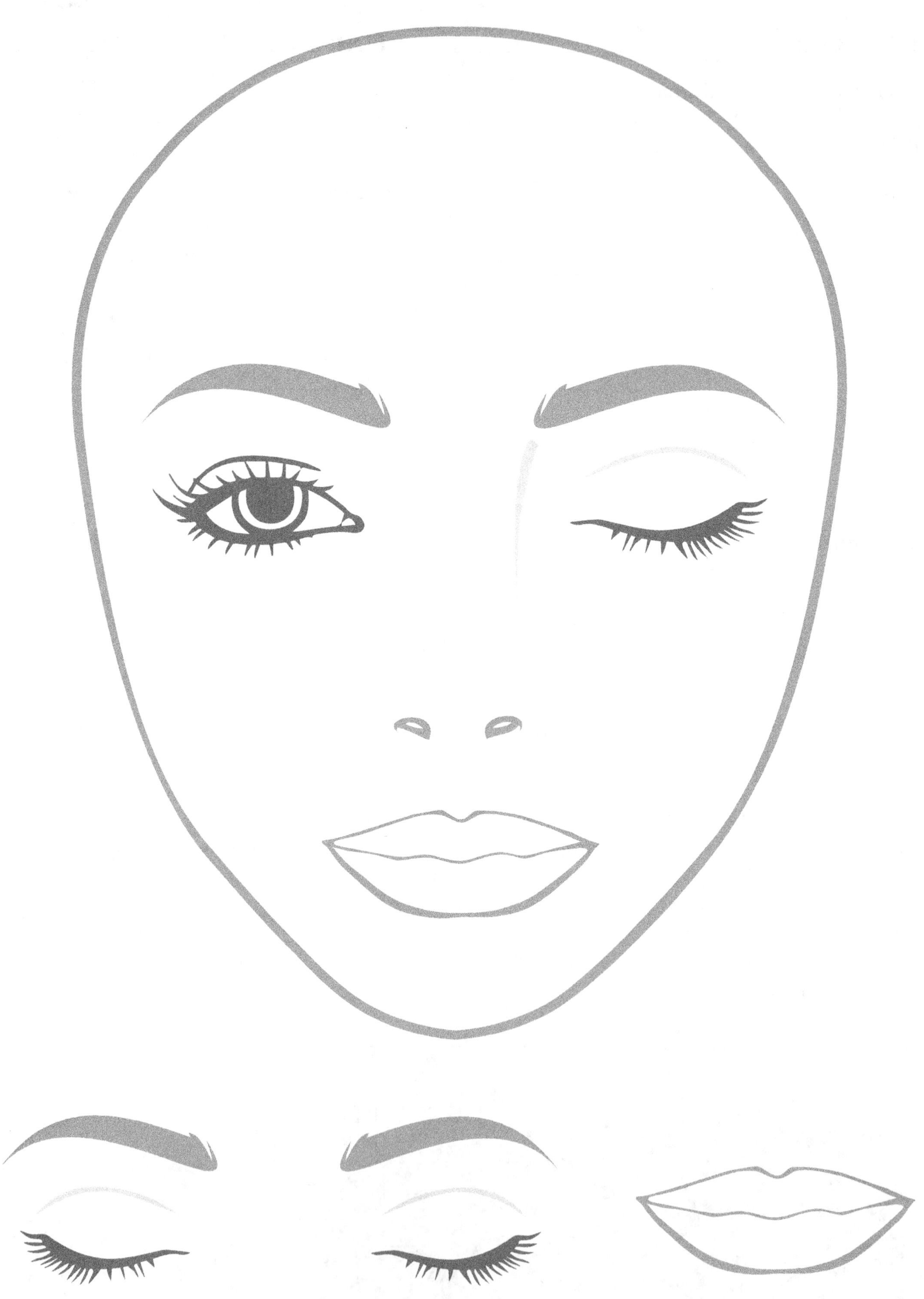

LOOK NAME ______________________ FOR: ______________________

◯ Daytime   ◯ Evening

FACE

Moisturizer

Concealer

Primer

Foundation

Powder

Contour

Highlight/Blush

EYES

Brows

Crease

LIPS

Liner

Eyelid

Mascara

Lip Color

Liner

Gloss

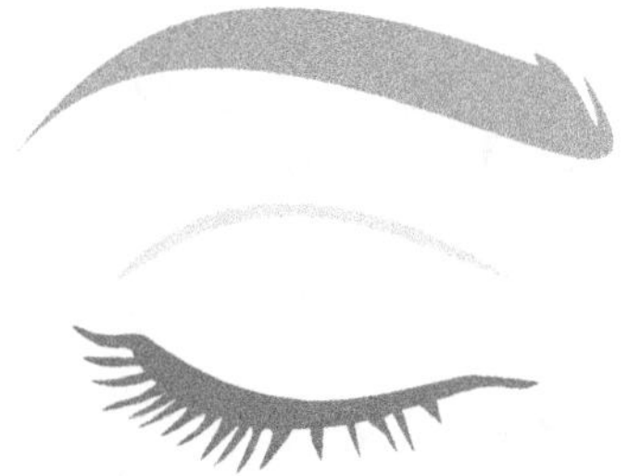
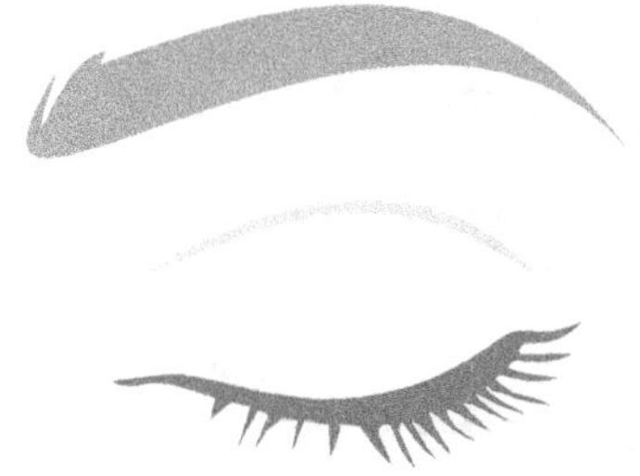
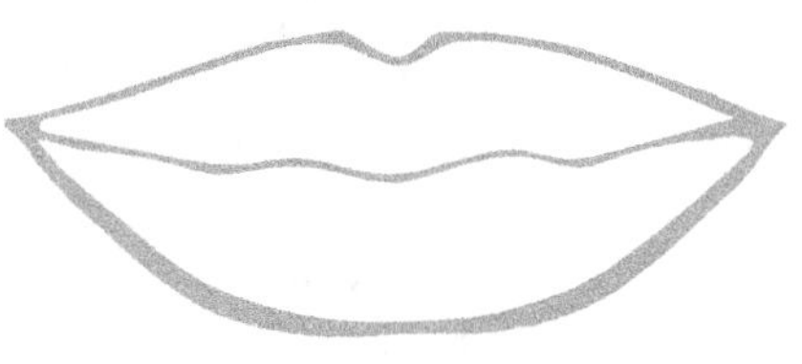

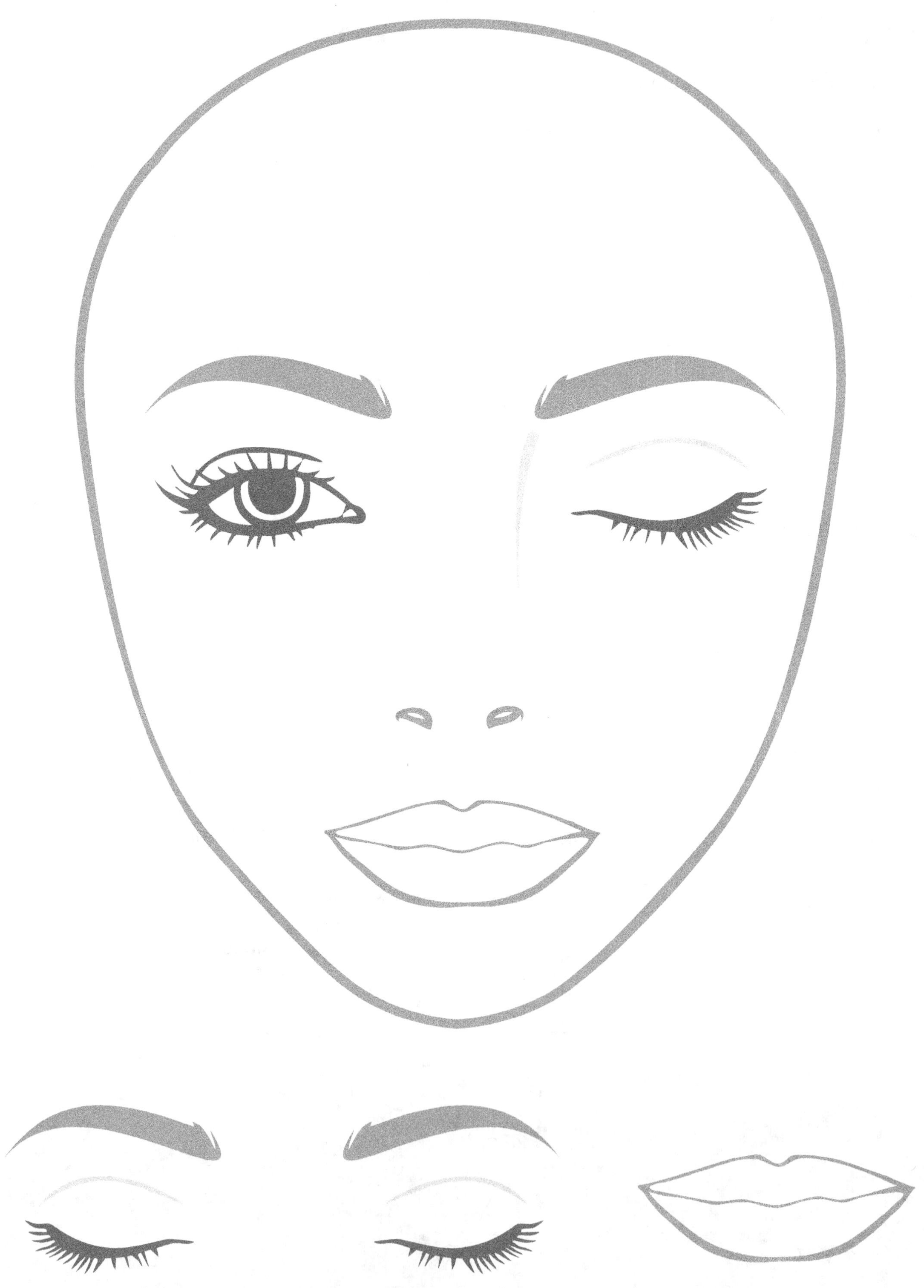

LOOK NAME ________________________________   **FOR:** ________________________________

◯ Daytime   ◯ Evening

FACE

Moisturizer

____

Primer

____

Powder

____

Highlight/Blush

____

Concealer

____

Foundation

____

Contour

____

EYES

Brows

____

Eyelid

____

Liner

____

Crease

____

Mascara

____

LIPS

Liner

____

Lip Color

____

Gloss

____

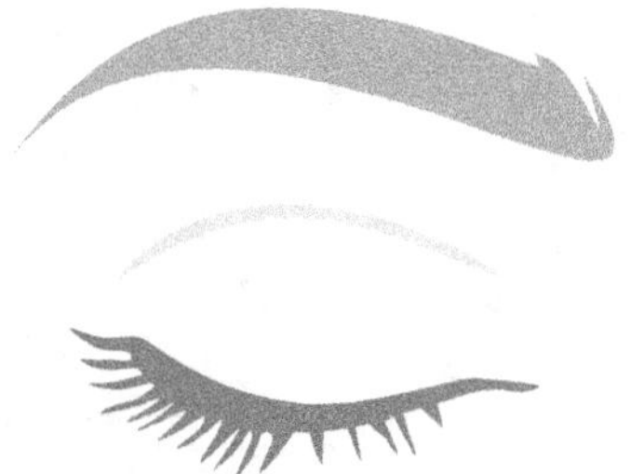

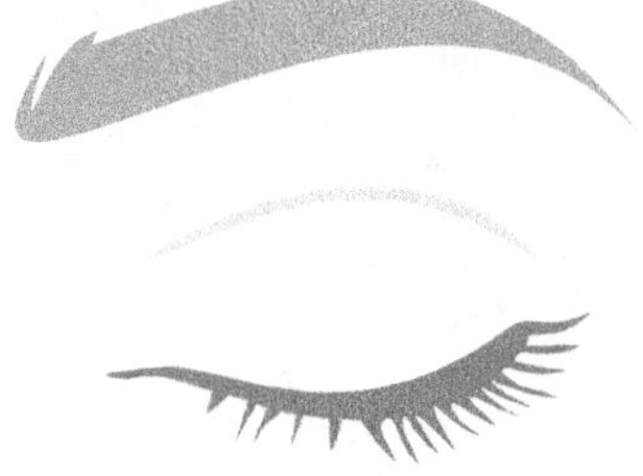

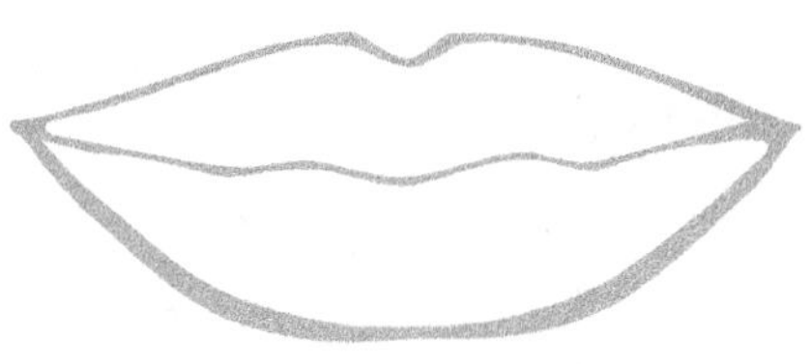